Medical Cannabis
Preparing for Oklahoma's Dispensaries

By
Christina Shifflett
The Green Nurse Educator

Medical Cannabis: Preparing for Oklahoma's Dispensaries

Copyright 2024 by Christina Shifflett
All rights reserved

Printed in the United States of America

Thank you for buying an authorized edition of this book and for complying with copyright laws by not reproducing, scanning, or distributing any part of it in any form without permission.

ISBN: 979-8-9900749-6-5 (Paperback)
ISBN: 979-8-9900749-7-2 (Large Print)
Library of Congress Control Number: 2024912455

First Edition: December 2024

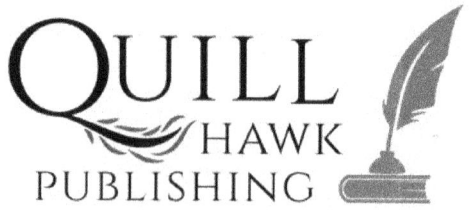

Quill Hawk Publishing
Oklahoma City, OK

Dedication

This book is dedicated first and foremost to my late husband, Will Shifflett. Without his love and support, I would not have started the journey to becoming a cannabis nurse educator. Before meeting Will, I had not given much thought to cannabis as a plant or medicine, but Will was such a huge cannabis supporter that he helped me see it as a viable treatment option. Will had experienced cannabis while growing up in California. He used to tell me the story of how he watched his friend's mom go through chemo treatments, losing weight rapidly and experiencing very low energy levels. She learned about cannabis and decided to give it a try. Will said the difference was startling; she was able to gain back some of the weight she lost and had more energy. Since that moment, Will had a newfound respect for cannabis as a medicine and began learning as much as he could about the plant. When I met Will, he was incredibly hopeful that medicinal cannabis would become federally legal so research could be completed specifically related to autism. The healthcare journey that my late husband embarked upon once they had received the autism diagnosis for my stepson was a hard one. Getting answers proved to be trial and error, an experience shared by many with similar struggles. Will would often reflect with me on the changes he saw in my stepson with traditional medicines. The hope for people not to have to continuously deal with the negative side effects of the medicine they need to take to have active, healthy lives is what inspired Will and me to learn as much as we could about cannabis as a medicine.

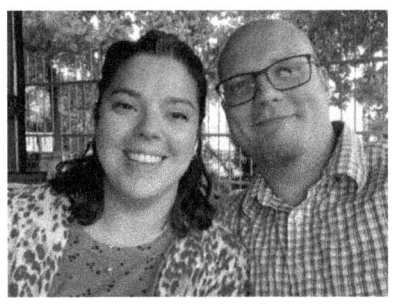

Photo 1 - Christina and Will

Table of Contents

Introduction and Goal of the Book	1
Commonly Used Terms and Definitions	3
Preparing to Go to the Dispensary	9
Consuming Cannabis	14
How Does Cannabis Interact with the Body?	23
Side Effects of Cannabis	26
Potency of Cannabis	32
New Consumers of Cannabis	36
Introduction to Cannabinoids, Flavonoids, and Terpenes	39
Cannabinoids	40
Terpenes	47
Flavonoids	72
Conclusion	79
Acknowledgments	81
About the author	83
Bibliography	84

Introduction and Goal of the Book

The Green Nurse Educator was created out of a desire to help everyday people understand more about cannabis and what effects it may have on the body.

The world of cannabis is constantly evolving as more and more research is being done on and with the cannabis plant. The amount of research, opinion, and conjecture surrounding cannabis that is readily available on the internet and social media can be overwhelming to wade through. The information in this booklet is intended to help simplify things.

After reading this book, you will have a basic understanding of the compounds inside the cannabis plant, what they could potentially be used for, the different types of cannabis products that are available and how they can be consumed or applied. While you are reading, keep in mind that the cannabis industry has been around in some shape or form for many centuries. In spite of this it has been actively researched for only a relatively short amount of time. For the better part of the previous century, cannabis has been classified as a Schedule I Drug according to the Food and Drug Administration (FDA). Schedule I drugs are classified as "Drugs, substances, or chemicals…with no currently accepted medical use and a high potential for abuse."[1] Because of the legal status of the plant and the restrictions in place, the research that could be done on the plant had to take place at only one university, which greatly decreased the number of studies that could be done on cannabis as a medicine.

The 2018 Farm Bill brought about some easing of the restrictions, allowing other companies to research cannabis as medicine and (among other things) for research to be done on more varieties of cannabis products.

Currently, research into cannabis as a medication is still in its infancy. The research that we have from before the 2018 Farm Bill generally came from studies that involved only a small number of participants, had time frames that were quite short, and had research questions that looked at the negative (applications for research on what cannabis *could* help with were not usually approved) and the cannabis that was studied could only come from a single growing facility. All of these factors combined do not give us an accurate representation or a complete understanding of the plant. Research since the Farm Bill gives us more information with each study that is published, but still there are roadblocks to navigate.

Hopefully in the near future, when cannabis is removed from its Schedule I status, more research will be completed.

Commonly Used Terms and Definitions

- Bong – a glass water pipe that is generally shaped like a beaker or a cup. This allows for water to filter the cannabis smoke before it is inhaled.
- Butane Hash Oil (BHO) – a potent cannabis concentrate made by dissolving the compounds within the plant into a solvent, usually in a complex process involving butane.
- Bud – the slang term for the flowers of the cannabis plant.
- Cannabinoids – a class of chemical compounds in the cannabis plant that act on the endocannabinoid receptors in our bodies.
- Cannabis – refers to all parts of the *Cannabis sativa L.* plant.
- Chemovars – also called chemotypes, strains, and cultivars. A chemovar describes a specific blend of terpenes, cannabinoids, flavonoids, and other components that make up the plant.
- Concentrates – very strong substances made from dissolving the cannabis plant material into a solvent, such as butane, ethanol, or MCT (medium-chain triglycerides) oil. This method extracts the cannabis compounds (THC, CBD and/or other compounds) from the plant into the solvent.
- Dabs/Dabbing – slang words for consuming cannabis concentrates.
- Dry herb vape – a device that is used to consume the dried flower of the cannabis plant. This device heats the flower without burning the material, vaporizing the plant. These vapes come in various sizes, from small handheld devices that are discrete to larger tabletop devices that look like a kitchen appliance.

- Edibles/Medibles – refers to cookies, brownies, cakes, drinks etc. that are prepared with cannabis for eating or drinking.
- Endocannabinoid – cannabinoids that are created by the body, such as 2-Arachidonoylglycerol (2-AG) and Anandamide (AEA).[2]
- Endocannabinoid system – "A signalling pathway that is found in the central nervous (CNS) and peripheral nervous systems (PNS) and immune pathways. This system is comprised of multiple receptors that, when activated…affect neurotransmitter release and subsequently influences a number of physiological factors such as immune response, cardiovascular function, bone development, digestion and metabolism, as well as several other process including wake/sleep cycles, learning, pain response, and regulation of stress and appetite."[3]
- Entourage effect – the suggested positive contribution (e.g. decreased pain or inflammation) that occurs when the whole plant is consumed. You would not get the entourage effect if the cannabis product that is being consumed has been isolated to extract only one type of compound. For example, if consuming CBD oil isolate, you would not get the effects of THC or any of the other multiple compounds in cannabis.
- First pass effect – the phenomenon in which a drug gets metabolized at a specific location in the body that results in a reduced concentration of the active drug upon reaching its site of action or the systemic circulation, most often associated with the liver.[4] Essentially, when a drug is swallowed it begins to be digested and is absorbed through the liver. As it "first passes" through the liver, the drug breaks down into a different compound. With Δ-9-THC it breaks down into 11-OH-THC when it goes through the liver, which is a more potent compound than Δ-9-THC is. This is

why there are far more stories of people taking too many edibles and "greening out" (experiencing the negative side effects of too much THC).
- Flavonoids – responsible for the color and aroma of plants. They also attract pollinators, protect from UV light and act as antimicrobial agents.
- Full spectrum – a full-spectrum extract includes a variety of cannabinoids, terpenes and sometimes even additional plant lipids.[5]
- GABA (Gamma-Aminobutyric Acid) – GABA is the most common inhibitory neurotransmitter in your central nervous system. Inhibitory neurotransmitters prevent or block chemical messages and decrease the stimulation of nerve cells in your brain. GABA is known for producing a calming effect. It is thought to play a major role in controlling nerve cell hyperactivity associated with anxiety, stress and fear.[4]
- Hash – short for hashish, a cannabis resin from the top of the plant, used for recreational and medicinal consumption.
- Hemp – a variety of cannabis grown for its fiber. It is non-psychoactive, meaning it does not affect the brain like high tetrahydrocannabinol (THC) cultivators can.
- Indica – the popular name for the *Cannabis indica* species of cannabis. Generally originated in the Middle East and Asia and includes both the famous Kush and Afghan lineages. Indica generally refers to cannabis cultivars that have a more sedating and calming high.
- Joint – a rolled cannabis cigarette, also known as a spliff, reefer, blunt, etc.
- Kief – a collected amount of trichomes (see definition) that have been separated from the rest of the cannabis flower. The kief can be used in several different ways such as adding it into your baking recipes as well as mixed into dried cannabis flower to be inhaled.

- Monoterpene – a chemical structure of the cannabis plant that has ten carbon atoms. Monoterpenes are a part of the terpenes group.[7]
- Phytocannabinoid – cannabinoids that come from a natural plant source, such as CBD and THC.
- Potency – refers to the strength of cannabis and is usually measured by the amount of THC within the plant.
- Purity – describes the ratio of compound within a product. I.e., how much THC/CBD/CBG is in a product and also refers to the absence of additives and chemicals.
- Sativa – the popular name for the *Cannabis Sativa* species of the cannabis plant. In general, they originated outside of the Middle East and Asia and include cultivars that are from areas such as South America, the Caribbean, Africa, and Thailand. Sativa also generally refers to cannabis cultivars that will have an uplifting and energizing effect on people.
- Sesquiterpene – a chemical structure of the cannabis plant with fifteen carbon atoms. Sesquiterpenes are a part of the terpenes group.
- Shatter – a transparent form of concentrated cannabis that, when cold, resembles an amber-colored glass. When it breaks apart, it "shatters".
- Schedule I drug – Schedule I drugs, substances, or chemicals are defined as drugs with no currently accepted medical use and a high potential for abuse. Some examples of Schedule I drugs are: heroin, lysergic acid diethylamide (LSD), marijuana (cannabis), 3,4-methylenedioxymethamphetamine (ecstasy), methaqualone and peyote.[1]
- Terpenes – aromatic oils secreted from oil glands called trichomes. They have a variety of characteristics, including flavor, smell, effects and medicinal potential. Terpenes are further classified by the number of atoms

and their arrangement. Examples of the different classifications of terpenes are monoterpenes, tetraterpenes, sesquiterpenes, and diterpenes to name a few.
- Tetrahydrocannabinol – the primary psychedelic compound, in cannabis that is responsible for the "high" effects. Also known as THC.
- Tincture – a liquid cannabis extract that is usually dosed with a dropper and is made using either alcohol or vegetable glycerine.
- Trichomes – a small hair or other outgrowth from the epidermis of the plant, typically unicellular and glandular. In cannabis plants, the trichomes are microscopic structures that typically look like really small light posts leaning one way or the other. The trichomes can be sticky with oil residue, which is where the cannabinoids and terpenes are stored inside of the plant.
- Triterpenoid – a chemical structure of the cannabis plant with 30 carbon atoms. Triterpenoids are a part of the terpenes group.
- Vape pen – a pen sized portable vaporizer that can be used with cannabis oil, wax, shatter, or flower.
- Vaporizer/Vaping – uses electricity to heat and evaporate cannabis without the combustion of flames. There are multiple types of vaporizing devices, ranging from handheld to tabletop versions.
- Wax – a form of cannabis concentrate that is similar to shatter but is more pliable, like traditional bees' wax.
- 2018 Farm Bill – In December of 2018, the 2018 Farm Bill was signed into Federal law. It removed hemp, defined as cannabis (*Cannabis sativa L.*) and derivatives of cannabis with extremely low concentrations of the psychoactive compound Δ-9-tetrahydrocannabinol (THC) (no more than 0.3% THC on a dry weight basis),

from the definition of marijuana in the Controlled Substances Act (CSA).[8]

Preparing to Go to the Dispensary

Cannabis Laws in the State of Oklahoma

Before going to a dispensary there are several laws to be aware of. Every state with a medical cannabis program has developed its own set of rules and regulations regarding cannabis use as well as what amounts of cannabis patients are allowed to have on hand. The list of qualifying symptoms or disease processes that cannabis can be used for is also going to be different depending on what state you live in. In Oklahoma, "A medical marijuana license must be recommended according to the accepted standards a reasonable and prudent physician would follow when recommending or approving any medication."[9] What this means is that the providers who recommend medical marijuana licensing in the state of Oklahoma consider the relevant research available on cannabis as well as the affecting symptoms the patient has when deciding if the license would be granted. Similarly to how doctors prescribe all their prescription medications.

When applying for a medical marijuana license in the state of Oklahoma, you have several different options; there are businesses online that provide full services (from provider recommendation to submission to the Oklahoma Medical Marijuana Association [OMMA]), businesses that provide easier access to medical professionals for the recommendation (generally online but can be in person) and then traditional primary care providers who also provide medical marijuana recommendations. Fees are associated with each option and discounts are available depending on the type of insurance a person has.

Within the state of Oklahoma, there are different types of licenses that a patient can apply for:

- Adult two-year license,
- Adult short-term license, up to 60 days
- Adult caregiver license for either adult or pediatric patients, up to 2 years, or
- Minor (0-17 years) license, up to 2 years.[10, 11]

If you are visiting an out-of-state dispensary, be sure to read up on cannabis laws specific to the state you are in. Some states offer reciprocity for medical marijuana licenses valid in your home state. Reciprocity means you would show them your Oklahoma medical marijuana license and would be allowed to purchase cannabis from their medical dispensaries just as if you had a medical marijuana license from that state.

Cannabis Limits in Oklahoma

It is incredibly important to know the limits of how much cannabis any one person may possess in your state. Having more than the limit of cannabis can expose a person to legal action and fees. As of early 2024, people who have medical marijuana cards in the state of Oklahoma may possess at any given time:

- Up to 3 oz of marijuana on their person,
- 6 mature plants and their harvested flowers,
- 6 seedling plants,
- 1 oz of concentrated cannabis,
- 8 oz total in their residence,
- 72 oz total of edible marijuana, and
- 72 oz total of topical marijuana.[11, 12]

Items Needed to Go to the Dispensary

When going to the dispensary, make sure to take your medical marijuana license. While dispensaries will store your information on their systems, legally, you must have your card with you to purchase cannabis from any dispensary. It is best practice to carry your medical marijuana card with you whenever you have cannabis in your car or on your person so that it can be shown readily when asked. A typical Oklahoma dispensary has its shop set up so that those without a medical marijuana card can come in and browse non-THC-related items while having the medical cannabis products in another room that only license holders may enter.

Due to federal banking regulations, not every store will be able to accept a card (debit or credit) for payment of cannabis products. These laws are actively being changed and new proposed laws are being brought up consistently, knowing this may change in the future. Most stores will typically have an ATM on site so that you can get cash there. Some stores will also have a handheld machine that acts as a mini-ATM, so you can swipe your card to pay for your purchases. These handheld machines act exactly like an ATM, be aware they will have charges associated with their use.

Know Before You Go

The information that is currently available surrounding cannabis can sometimes be overwhelming. Then there is also the question of who knows this

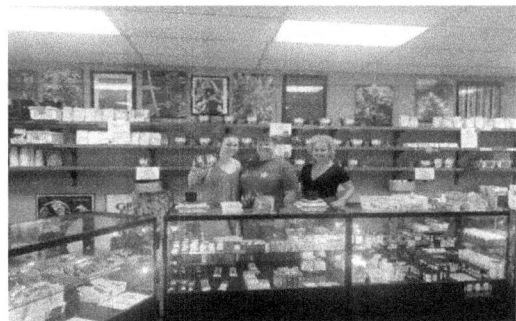

Photo 2 - Budtenders at Natural Remedies MMJ in Enid, Oklahoma

information best or who has the most accurate and up-to-date information. Aside from researching the Oklahoma Medical Marijuana Authority website (OMMA), the regulating body in Oklahoma, your cannabis nurse and dispensary budtenders should be your next go-to for all questions related to cannabis!

Budtenders are going to be an excellent resource within the dispensary. However, standard credentialing for budtenders has just come into effect at the beginning of 2024, so don't be afraid to ask them all the questions as well as do your own research. Not only will they have information about the types of cannabis that are sold at the dispensary, but they should also be able to give anecdotal information about what other people are buying. Typically, budtenders help one customer at a time, which means patients get their undivided attention. Write down any questions you may have before going to the dispensary and then use that as a conversation starter. If the questions you have are too complex for a budtender, they should also be able to recommend a healthcare professional who would be able to help answer those questions. The Green Nurse Educator is one of those healthcare professionals who can help with complex medical and cannabis questions.

When you are at the dispensary, it is a good idea to ask the budtender to see the Certificate of Analysis (COA) for the product that you are buying. It is an entirely appropriate question to ask and should be within easy reach for the budtender to pass along to you. The COA may be on hand in paper format, as shown in Photo 3, and it may also be in digital format on the website for that cannabis product. A major red flag for a dispensary is if a customer receives resistance when asking to see the COA.

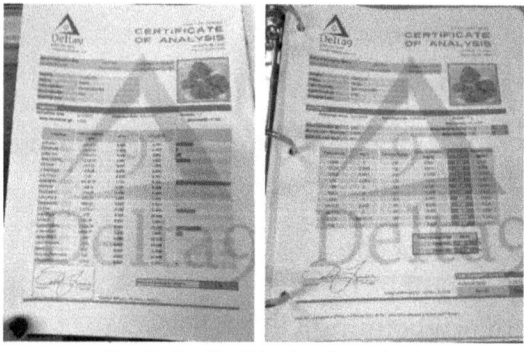

Photo 3 - Certificate of Analysis

The COA will tell you exactly what levels of terpenes and cannabinoids are within the product. Though a COA can be a bit data-heavy to read, it can be an incredibly valuable tool when looking at cannabis as a medication. As testing for different cannabinoids becomes more refined, we will be able to know *exactly* what types of compounds we are putting into our bodies while consuming this cannabis.

As a reminder, every state is going to have different limits on how much consumable cannabis you can purchase in one trip — there is no cannabis wholesaler. Your budtenders should be aware of the limits within the state and should not sell you more than is legal. That said, always do your research before going to the dispensary as well as ask questions during your visit.

Another reminder that if you do not have your unexpired medical marijuana card with you when you go to the dispensary, you will not be able to go into the portion of the store that is dedicated to consumable cannabis with high THC, nor will you be able to purchase any THC. Some dispensaries will sell CBD-related products in a different room accessible to the public (age restrictions may apply).

Consuming Cannabis

Routes of Consumption

By now, you have received some information on how to get your card, the laws in Oklahoma, and what to bring with you to the dispensary. Next, you are faced with MANY choices in how to consume cannabis. If you've never consumed cannabis before, it can be a daunting choice. Below, you will find information about the types of cannabis products available, the different methods of consuming cannabis, and then in the next section, we will go into how quickly or slowly those routes will take effect on the body.

Oral:

The first route of consumption we're going to talk about is consuming cannabis via the oral route. There are gummies, tinctures, oils, pills, and edibles. Edibles can be an excellent choice to try out the first time as the taste can be masked by the food it is in, but make sure to read the dosage instructions when going the edible route. Any consumable cannabis (or any type of consumable, medicine, or food) that is swallowed and will go through your digestive tract is considered the oral route.

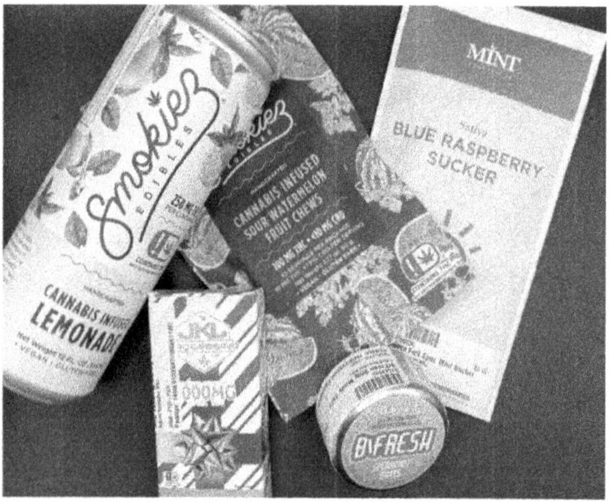

Photo 4 - Examples of cannabis consumed via the oral route.

Tinctures are listed in the oral category as well as in the sublingual/buccal category because they can be consumed both ways. If a tincture is mixed in with a drink and consumed that way, it will go through the digestive tract and is considered the oral route. However, if the tincture is held in the mouth (under the tongue or against the cheek) until the medicine is fully absorbed, that is considered the sublingual/buccal route.

Inhalation:

The next method of cannabis consumption to discuss is the inhalation route, such as traditional smoking, vaping, and dabbing. When cannabis is inhaled in this manner, all the cannabinoids and terpenes are absorbed through the lungs.

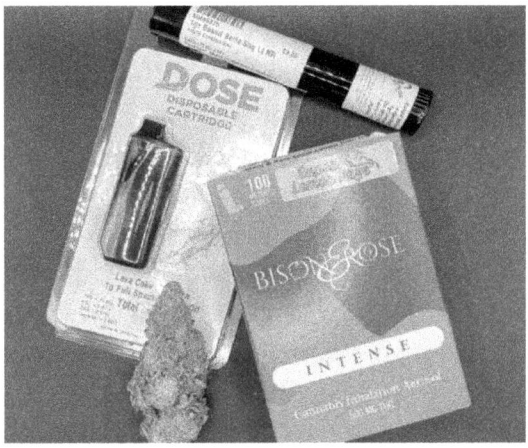

Photo 5 - Examples of cannabis consumed via the inhalation route.

There have been some amazing strides made in the way we can consume cannabis, such that there are even inhalers available for those who do not want to smoke or vape. There are even some that are quite small and discreet. The inhalation route is perhaps the most common way of consuming cannabis as well as the most traditional. However, inhaling cannabis can pose a risk to the lungs simply due to the fact that when smoking or vaping, you're exposing your lungs to an irritant that they might not otherwise have. Care should be taken with any medicine that is absorbed through the lungs. Consult with your cannabis nurse if you have any concerns about cannabis and your lungs.

Sublingual:

The sublingual (under the tongue) and buccal (inside the cheek) routes of cannabis consumption are not often recognized as distinct from the oral route, but they are actually quite different. When taking cannabis (or any other medicine) via the sublingual or buccal

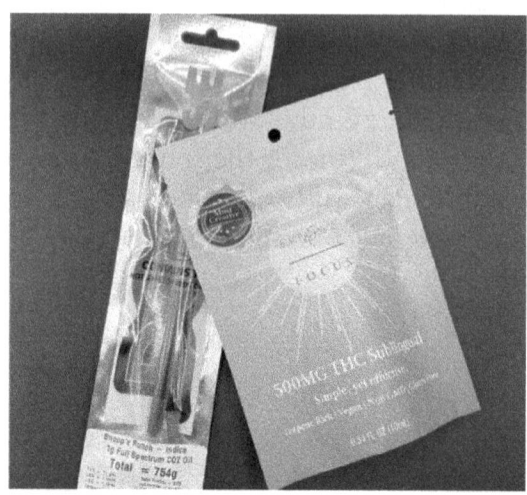

Photo 6 - Examples of cannabis consumed via the sublingual or buccal route.

route, the medicine is not swallowed. If the medicine is swallowed, then it will go through the digestive tract and take a bit longer for the medicine to be absorbed properly. However, if the medicine is absorbed under the tongue or through the cheek lining, it takes effect far more quickly. Part of the reason that there aren't more sublingual products available is that taking cannabis via the sublingual or buccal route can sometimes be difficult to do. This stems from the fact that a sublingual medicine is most easily made in a tincture format, and a tincture is usually made with high-grade alcohol, at least 80 proof. The end product can be quite uncomfortable to hold in your mouth for very long as it is abrasive to the tissues there. Little pills that dissolve under the tongue can also be made into a cannabis product, but the breakdown of the pill under the tongue can be quite bitter.

Topical:

The last method of cannabis consumption that we will discuss is the topical route. A topical medication refers to any oil, cream, or lotion that is meant to be applied to and absorbed by the skin. For a person inexperienced with

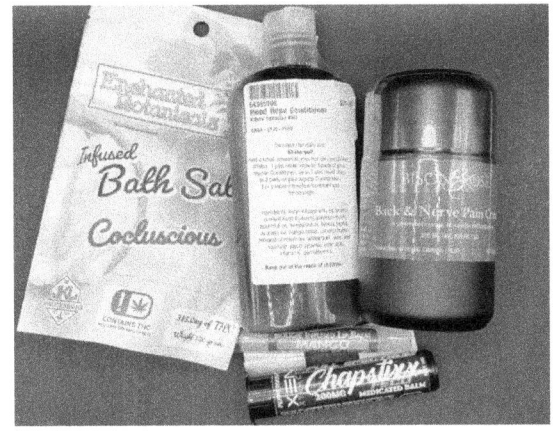

Photo 7 - Topical cannabis products

cannabis, starting with a topical product can be a low-risk option. Some medicinal marijuana patients prefer topical products over other products because they can put it right on the area that is affecting them. Another benefit to applying cannabis to the skin is that the person using the cream is very unlikely to feel any of the traditional effects that come with consuming elevated levels of THC (more about the side effects of THC in an upcoming section). For a person dealing with chronic conditions that affect their daily life, having a method of treating that chronic condition without decreasing their ability to function in social and work settings can be invaluable.

In summary, there are several different ways to consume cannabis. The variety and availability of different cannabis compounds in Oklahoma dispensaries is amazing to see. This allows you, the consumer, to tailor your medication regimen in such a way that it maximizes your energy during the day and supports your sleep at night, as well as helping you with your symptoms. Here is a short list of the different methods of cannabis consumption.

- Oral
  - Gummies
  - Tinctures
  - Edibles
  - Oils
- Inhalation
  - Aerosol
  - Vaping
  - Smoking
  - Dabs
- Sublingual/buccal
  - Tinctures
  - Tablets
- Topical
  - Creams and lotions
  - Oils
  - Suppositories*

*Suppositories, although more a part of the oral/enteral pathway, are classified in the topical category as well as this is typically how they are presented within the dispensary itself.

Times of Onset and Length of Duration

When taking cannabis for medical purposes, the timing of the onset of the medication is quite important. Patients taking cannabis as medication do not want to experience negative effects that could come with either not having enough medication in their system to deal with their chronic conditions or having too much medication in their system, leading to the traditional "high" symptoms (such as dizziness, paranoia, dry mouth, etc.). Understanding how and when to take cannabis in such a way as to provide the maximum amount of coverage is paramount. In the next sections, we're going to go over the different routes for cannabis medicine, how quickly they will begin to take effect, and how long they can generally last in the body.

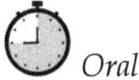 *Oral*

When consuming cannabis via the oral route, you can expect to feel effects around 45 minutes from the time you consumed the cannabis product. The oral route includes anything that is swallowed and goes through the entire digestive system. A quick reminder - the oral route includes pills, gummies, candies, drinks, chocolates and others. Variables such as what the cannabis is cooked into and how regularly the patient's digestive tract moves can result in shorter or longer times between consumption and the time the effect is felt. During the process of digestion, cannabis components are broken down by the liver into secondary metabolites (compounds) or inactive compounds that can sometimes be more potent than the primary compound.[13] An example of this would be how THC starts out as Δ9-THC in a gummy or chocolate but then is converted to 11-hydroxy-THC by the liver. The process of cannabis (or any other medicine) being broken down through the digestive tract/the liver is known as first-pass metabolism.[4]

Any medicine, including cannabis, when consumed via the oral route is going to begin having an effect anywhere from 30 to 45 minutes after consumption. Times may vary with onset as digestion plays a big role in this process. Cannabis is also more easily digested in foods that contain a lot of fat, as cannabis binds readily with fat.[14] Cannabis is naturally fat soluble, which means eating cannabis with foods higher in fats, such as peanut butter, oil, or butter, will help the cannabinoids and terpenes bind and absorb easily. There are ways to make cannabis a water-soluble product (meaning it dissolves in water instead of needing a fat to bind with)[14, 15] that is popular for cannabis drink products and cannabis powders.

Remember: when cannabis is consumed via the oral route, it has to go through the whole digestive system to eventually be broken down into its inactive components.[16] This process can last between 6 and 12 hours, depending on how quickly your digestive system moves. Accidentally consuming too much THC orally may lead to uncomfortable side effects that can last for up to 12 hours.

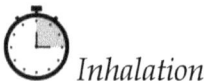 *Inhalation*

Inhaling cannabis has been a long-standing tradition among cannabis consumers, mostly by smoking cannabis in a joint, bong (see definitions list), or pipe. As time has gone by, cannabis has also become available in vaping and aerosol formats. Cannabis can be vaped through various apparatuses such as vape pens or dry herb vapes, which can be especially attractive if discreet use is important. Recently, cannabis has also become available in aerosol form, similar to an asthma inhaler. Cannabis consumed via the inhalation route will take effect more rapidly than most of the other cannabis consumption methods as it crosses into the bloodstream readily through the lining of the mouth and lungs. You'll begin to feel an effect within 2-15 minutes after inhaling. If you're not used to inhaling cannabis, low and slow is the way to trial it out. Take one puff and wait 15 minutes to see how it affects your body and symptoms.[14, 15] If you don't receive the desired effect, take another puff at 15 minutes and repeat as needed. The effects of inhaling cannabis come on quicker, but they also begin to decrease quickly as compared to the oral route. Generally, the effects of inhaling cannabis can last up to 6 hours in our bodies but can begin to fade within the first hour.[17] Each person's unique metabolism will help the THC cycle out of their system at different rates.[17]

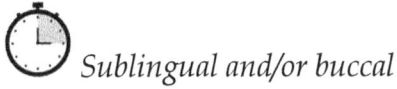 *Sublingual and/or buccal*

Sublingual means to let the medicine dissolve under the tongue,[18] while buccal means that the medicine should be dissolved in the cheek.[19] The sublingual and buccal routes of administration can be especially useful for individuals who have difficulty swallowing, such as patients in hospice care. Neither of these routes is truly intended to be swallowed but rather allowed to be held under the tongue or inside the cheek until it has been all absorbed. Tinctures, Rick Simpson Oil, and dissolvable tablets are some examples of sublingual and buccal cannabis products. Medicines given via the sublingual or buccal route should begin to take effect within 10 to 15 minutes.[14] The sublingual or buccal route could be the preferred method for giving medicine to a person who is unable to swallow effectively, as sublingual and buccal medicines do not need to be swallowed to begin working.[20] Cannabis preparations designed to be given via the sublingual or buccal route are generally made with high-grade alcohol, food-grade glycerine, or water-soluble powders. Products made with high-grade alcohol are called tinctures and can be really harsh on the soft tissue lining of the mouth. The tincture can be diluted with a bit of water or another beverage, but then it will most likely be swallowed and, therefore, not provide sublingual or buccal timeframes and benefits. Products made with food-grade glycerine are called glycerites and are not generally found in dispensaries but would be incredibly easy to make in the home. Lastly, water-soluble powders can be made into small pills or pastilles that can be held under the tongue or in the cheek to dissolve. Unfortunately, making water-soluble powders can be a complex process and might not be as easy to make oneself.

Medicines that are taken via the sublingual or buccal route tend to stay active in the system for 6-8 hours.[14]

 *Topical*

Applying cannabis in a topical form can be incredibly useful for people dealing with a multitude of different symptoms. When applying cannabis topically, it does not go through the liver (first-pass effect) and will not break down into 11-hydroxy-THC (the more potent form of THC) as it does when cannabis is eaten (or taken orally). Topical cannabis products are gels, creams, sprays, and lotions—anything that goes on to the skin really. They go directly on or over the site that is having an issue. Topicals can start having an effect in 30 minutes to 2 hours and can typically last in the body for 1 to 8 hours.[14] This route is incredibly useful in helping maintain normal joint and skin health.[14, 15] The benefit of applying cannabis topically is that the medicine is going directly on the area that is having an issue (pain, inflammation, etc.). This means that the compounds within the cannabis cream will not have to travel as far to connect with the ECS receptors that are closest to the site of injury (more about this in the next section). As mentioned before, the cannabis cream will not go through the liver and will not cross the blood-brain barrier to cause the traditional "high" that is generally associated with high THC cannabis. This makes topical products the perfect starter product for anyone trying cannabis as a medicine.

How Does Cannabis Interact with the Body?

This section is packed with information related to how cannabis interacts with the body and perhaps a bit more clinical. It is, however, crucial to go over the basics of how cannabis interacts with your receptors to understand how to choose your medicine. This will be a broad overview of a complex topic that is still evolving as we learn more.

Recent research has shown that all humans and animals have a signaling system within our bodies that directly interacts with cannabis compounds. This is called the endocannabinoid system (ECS), which is a lipid signaling system in our bodies that consists of cannabinoid receptors, the endogenous ligands that bind to them, and the enzymes that control their synthesis (creation) and degradation (breakdown).[14] The receptors that are currently being studied are the cannabinoid receptor 1 (CB1) and the cannabinoid receptor 2 (CB2). There is also a signaling pathway called the transient receptor potential vanilloid 1 (TRPV1) that is being studied as it helps to modulate the way our brain interprets pain.[14]

Our bodies receive help from the ECS to regulate hormonal processes and produce their own endocannabinoids ("endo" meaning from within). The two most well-known endocannabinoids are arachidonoyl ethanolamine (AEA) and 2-arachidonoylglycerol (2-AG). These receptors are created and broken down through amazingly complex cellular pathways within the body.[14] The minute intricacies of the interactions between our ECS and the endocannabinoids from our bodies, much less the phytocannabinoids that come from cannabis and other plants, is beyond the scope of this booklet. However, there are multiple excellent explanations of this process available on the internet. The basic premise of the interaction is that the compounds within cannabis interact without ECS, prompting it to send signals further down their proper pathway (like telling the body to turn down the inflammation process once an injury has healed). You could almost think of our ECS as a series of light switches, and the phytocannabinoids switch them on or off depending on their original purpose.

The cannabinoids that we get from consuming cannabis are called phytocannabinoids. "Phyto" means related to plants. Cannabinoids that are absorbed into the body from plants in the form of foods, creams, or smokeable products (from the cannabis plant as well as other plants) are phytocannabinoids. We mainly think of cannabinoids as coming from cannabis, but they can also be found in many other plants, such as lavender and hops.

The receptors that interact with cannabis are spread throughout our bodies. CB1 receptors are thought to be mainly concentrated in the nervous system and brain but can also be found in the peripheral nervous system and peripheral tissues, such as cardiovascular, gastrointestinal, and reproductive tissues.[14] CB2 receptors that were previously thought to only be located in the peripheral nervous system can also be found in immune cells, such as leukocytes (a cell a part of our immune system), and they are also found in the central nervous system.[15] It was previously thought that the receptors were only within certain areas of the body, but as research has progressed, scientists are finding that the CB1 and CB2 receptors are scattered throughout the body and are expressed (meaning they cause an action) in areas only intermittently or as needed.[14] This is unique from other receptors that are only ever "on" or "off."

When learning about the science of cannabinoid receptors, it's worth mentioning the location of the opioid receptors. The exact method of interaction between cannabinoid and opioid receptors is still unclear, but research has shown that these receptors DO interact with one another and have been shown to help increase the effectiveness of pain management.[14] These two receptors are located fairly close to each other on the synapse, where they normally reside, which could contribute to their interactions together.[21] There have been research studies examining the effect cannabis has on a person's mental and physical need for opioid medicines. These studies have generally shown that the consumption of cannabis has decreased the need for opioids by about 17% in those with chronic pain.[22] Continued research into cannabis has the potential to change the amount of pain medications people will need to take for their pain in the future.

For anyone taking opioids or any other medication that can cause respiratory depression, it is incredibly important to discuss your consumption methods with your provider and cannabis nurse. If multiple medications that decrease your ability to breathe effectively are taken together, the risk increases of that occurring. Why is this such an important topic to discuss when cannabis has not been shown to cause respiratory depression? The main reason for the discussion is that while cannabis might not cause respiratory depression, it does interact with opioids and anxiety medications, potentially causing them to have a stronger effect than normal, which could lead to respiratory depression. Breathing is vital to life, and we don't want anything to compromise that.

Side Effects of Cannabis

Side effects of cannabis are not often discussed at length due to the nature of the effects themselves. From a recreational standpoint, some of the effects that could be perceived as negative (i.e., disorientation or dizziness) can be purposely sought out by those who are consuming cannabis recreationally. Whereas from a medicinal standpoint, those effects that could inhibit a person's daily life (disorientation and/or dizziness) are seen as negative, and we try to avoid them. This section highlights the various side effects that are possible with cannabis, how to mitigate them, and what to do if you accidentally take too much THC.

If you are new to the cannabis world, you may or may not be familiar with the side effects that cannabis can have. However, you will have likely watched a movie or show that had a "typical stoner" character. Generally, this character is someone who is dressed primarily for comfort in oversized clothing; they're slow moving, not intelligent and consistently not understanding the questions/conversations they're a part of. Even though a lot of movies have portrayed the "stoner" character, and it is quite accepted in society as such, someone consuming cannabis medicinally doesn't typically fit that character type.

According to the Mayo Clinic, cannabis has the potential to cause the following side effects:

- Headaches
- Dry mouth and dry eyes
- Light-headedness and dizziness
- Drowsiness and fatigue
- Nausea and vomiting
- Disorientation
- Hallucinations

- Increased heart rate
- Increased appetite
- Impaired attention, judgment, and coordination.[23]

These side effects may look mild (in comparison to the side effect list of some prescription medications) but they can be overwhelming, especially if the person dealing with these side effects is a first-time or new again consumer of cannabis. A person new to cannabis who experiences these side effects could very well decide that cannabis is not the medication for them and never receive the potential benefits of it as a medicine. This is why it is so incredibly important to start at a low dose of cannabis and increase it slowly.

To complicate matters, whether someone experiences side effects depends on several factors. These include prior cannabis consumption, the amount consumed, the method of consumption (e.g., edible vs. smoking), any medications (prescription or otherwise) taken that day, and the type and amount of food eaten before or during cannabis use. All of these can influence the side effects a person may experience. That's a lot of factors to balance out and a big part of why there are so many stories of people who had a difficult time during their first time-consuming cannabis. Cannabis side effects can be mild to moderate but have the potential to be quite uncomfortable if large doses are consumed. Side effects of cannabis can be so discomforting that the consumer might think they need to take themselves to an ER to be treated. In a previous section, we discussed the various times that it takes for cannabis to take effect on the body, depending on the type of cannabis that is consumed. Smoking or vaping allows for the quickest onset of symptom relief and can stop acting on the body within 30 mins to an hour, but when consuming an edible, it starts to take effect within 45 mins and can last within the body anywhere from 4 to 8 hours. That can make for an uncomfortable time frame for a novice consumer if they accidentally take too much THC.

Mitigating the side effects of cannabis

Not all of the side effects of cannabis are considered uncomfortable. Recreational consumers might be purposefully pursuing these side effects - the feeling of floating along with rose-colored glasses would be a great example here. When consuming medicinally the end goal is to take the least amount of THC needed to ease the symptoms while also still being able to interact with the public and social environment appropriately. The main way of mitigating the side effects of cannabis is to prevent the side effects from happening in the first place. Beginning with a low starting dosage and increasing slowly over several days is the best way to do this. Two other strategies to help keep the side effects down are by taking CBD alongside the THC and by taking care of your body. CBD is naturally going to help keep THC in check because they both compete for some of the same receptor sites. A good rule of thumb is to take at least double the amount of CBD as you do of THC. CBD has been studied multiple times and has been shown to have a protective effect against the negative side effects of THC. We'll discuss dosing considerations for cannabis in a later section.

What to do if you accidentally get too high

Research has shown that a person is more likely to experience potentially serious side effects at dosages over 50 mg.[24] However every person has a unique endocannabinoid system and will feel the side effects differently. When reviewing the literature regarding cannabis side effects, there are very few that can cause life-threatening situations. Even though the chance of experiencing life-threatening situations from cannabis is quite low, the person consuming the cannabis might have an illness or disease process that could become critical when cannabis is consumed. This same article goes on to say that regular consumption of high doses of cannabis can lead to cannabinoid hyperemesis syndrome (CHS). CHS is a condition characterized by cyclical bouts of vomiting that seem to be relieved by hot baths. These are just a few of the reasons why it is so important to have a conversation with your primary care provider and a cannabis nurse about your cannabis consumption before consuming.

There are several anecdotal ways to help deal with being "too high". They are anecdotal because the research has not yet been done to prove whether they work consistently, if at all. Cannabis consumers, however, have been swearing by them for years. Supposedly, if a person is too high, they can drink milk or chew on peppercorns (the seasoning) to help reduce the symptoms. Bear in mind of course, that getting a person who is too high to drink a glass of milk or to chew on some peppercorns might not be the easiest task to accomplish. Videos can be seen on social media of influencers trying out eating peppercorns while too high to see if it helps decrease the negative side effects. It seems like the taste and texture of the peppercorn might be what helps bring the person back to earth.

A method that is being researched is the consumption of CBD to control the side effects of THC.[25] Consuming CBD when too high is something that has been practiced for such a long time that it is part of cannabis culture. Habitually consuming CBD with your THC is a good way to help reduce the potential of having those side effects in the first place. If one finds themselves too high for comfort, taking a CBD gummy, smoking/vaping a CBD joint, or even applying CBD cream could help reduce the symptoms. Beyond taking CBD, the main thing to do for people who get too high is to manage whatever current symptoms they are experiencing. If they're really thirsty, have them hydrate (try to avoid caffeine or anything stimulating); if they're feeling disoriented or are overstimulated, help them get to a quieter/calmer area so they can relax; if they're really hungry, help them find some healthy snacks. It's important to note that during this time, the person who is too high is not able to operate heavy machinery, is unable to legally consent and should not make any important decisions during this time.

Confusing factors with side effects
The risk for negative side effects can be increased for a variety of reasons, and one of the major reasons could be due to the packaging of the cannabis products. Oklahoma cannabis laws mandate that

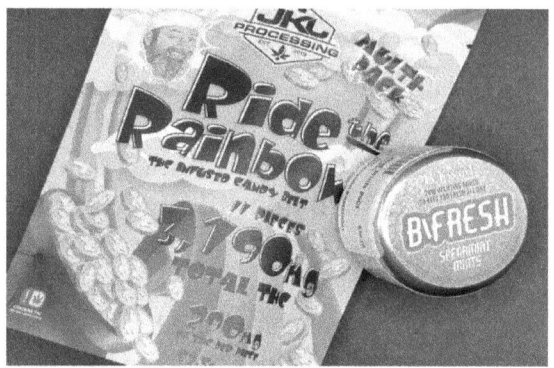

Photo 8 - Edibles of varying dosages

cannabis processors put the total milligrams of THC on the outside of the package to help reduce potential overdoses. However, sometimes, discerning the dosages per individual piece of the product can be challenging, depending on where the information is placed on the packaging. It is incredibly vital to know about the product you're going to try before buying it, as well as to take the time to look over the packaging while you're at the dispensary. Photo 8 shows an example of two different products that have vastly different dosages per individual piece. If a novice cannabis consumer picked up the gummies on the left side of Photo 8 and had one piece, they would be consuming 290 mg of THC, which is an astronomical amount of THC for someone who is not used to the effects of cannabis. Whereas the mints on the right side of Photo 8 have 2 mg of THC and are an excellent starting dose for someone who is new to cannabis. At such a low starting dose, the dosage can be increased gently and the chances of experiencing negative side effects would be lower. It is always good practice to start *low* and increase *slowly*.

It should be noted that if you are purchasing cannabis edibles, you need to store them properly. All cannabis products should be stored in a cool, dark place that is up and secure, away from anyone other than their intended consumer. Cannabis should also be stored in child-proof containers, as large doses of cannabis can have deleterious effects on young children.

Another reason to keep your edibles stored in a cool, dark location is to help preserve the original doses of the edible. Let's say that you recently picked up a package of cannabis gummies or chocolates but then forgot them in the car when it's warm out. The next time you get an edible from that package, they've all melted to some degree. Chocolates would definitely lose their shape and while some gummies might lose their shape as well, would they have melted enough that some of the cannabis extract has melted out as well? And once the edible is melted it's generally more difficult to reshape them than their worth. So, keeping your edibles stored properly can help you save money in the long run and preserve the integrity of the original dosage.

Potency of Cannabis

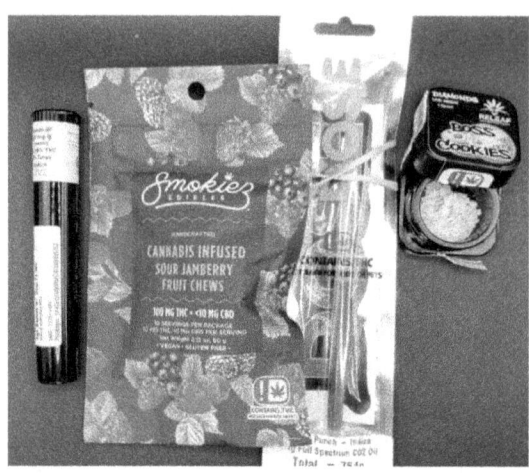

Photo 9 - From left to right the cannabis increases in potency.

When deciding what cannabis preparation to consume, it is important to take into consideration how potent the preparation might be as well as its intended purpose. Depending on the reason for taking cannabis, a patient might want to have a fast-acting cannabis, like a vape or aerosol, that they have with them throughout the day in case of breakthrough issues. That person might also take a longer-acting, slower-starting cannabis, like edibles, at regular intervals throughout the day. Photo 9 highlights the differences in potency levels among a variety of cannabis products. If a novice consumer started on the right side of Photo 9 by consuming diamonds on their first try, they are more likely to feel the negative side effects of cannabis than any health benefits. Whereas if a novice consumer starts with a joint or flower, they are less likely to experience the negative side effects of cannabis.

Since there are so many different ways to consume cannabis, not to mention the different things that you can make the cannabis plant into, it's good to know what the baseline or lowest potency product is so a novice cannabis consumer can start there. When we're discussing the potency of cannabis, we're looking at the type of product as well as the THC levels within each product. This could be slightly difficult to understand as there are so many different cultivars of cannabis with so many different THC levels. There is a subset population of cannabis consumers that like to grow their own plants, and some may be specifically growing cannabis to increase THC levels. For this portion of the chapter, we will first consider the different product types and not necessarily the THC percentage (that will be covered later). The cannabis plant/flower, as you would see it growing from the earth, would be considered our baseline potency level. This is primarily due to the fact that within the cannabis flower, you have so many different compounds that can provide health benefits aside from THC alone. This means that if you are consuming cannabis flower, the other compounds (cannabinoids and terpenes) will help to keep THC in check. The second reason is that anytime you make the cannabis flower into something else (such as edibles, diamonds, concentrates), you are concentrating and potentially isolating for individual compounds (like THC, CBD, CBG, etc.), which can increase the overall potency or strength of the end product. So, when deciding which cannabis product to start with, consider the fact that a smaller amount of concentrated product may have the same effect (if not more) than what you would expect from the cannabis flower.

According to the Journal of the Missouri State Medical Association, the average THC level in the cannabis plant has increased over 212% since the 1990s.[26] There are several reasons for this: First, cannabinoids and terpenes in the cannabis plant are the plant's natural defences against insects and animals. If there is a greater exposure to "predators" (insects) of the cannabis plant, THC levels might be higher to address the issue.[27] Another reason for higher levels of THC is the human component. People have been consuming cannabis to get high or help with health issues for a long time; some of them are specifically growing cannabis for higher THC levels. This is a great reason to develop a good relationship/rapport with your local budtender, as they will be able to help you choose a cultivar with THC levels that will help meet your needs. I have seen cannabis flowers in dispensaries local to me that have THC levels ranging from 11% to close to 30%. I am consistently astounded by the variety and ease of access that we Oklahomans have to cannabis. However, if you're new to cannabis, 30% THC could be too much to start out with. Remember, start low and go slow!

Higher potency cannabis has an increased chance of causing the negative side effects discussed previously. However, the length of time a person has been consuming cannabis is also a factor in whether they will experience side effects. An experienced cannabis consumer will also have developed a certain tolerance to the cannabis they are consuming and will need to periodically take breaks to bring their tolerances back down. Recent research showed that tolerance breaks occurring about every 30 days has the maximum benefit on the body,[28] but the length of the tolerance breaks is still subject to debate. While, for the occasional consumer, it takes about 21 days for THC to be completely cleared from the body, research suggests tolerance breaks can be as short as two days.[24] The CB1 receptors in the brain of chronic cannabis consumers are decreased during daily use but start to return to normal levels after just two days of abstinence from cannabis. This can be good news for those who take cannabis daily for their chronic conditions as they won't need to go too long without their preferred medication. Some patients rely heavily on cannabis to help control their chronic symptoms so taking extended breaks from cannabis could seem unfathomable or intolerable.

Another fact to consider when discussing the potency of cannabis is the age of the person consuming the cannabis. As we age our metabolism tends to slow down and medicines can have a bigger or more prolonged effect than the consumer is anticipating. Medications that pass through the liver, such as cannabis, can potentially give a 30% higher effect than the patient is expecting. As we age, our liver can potentially lose the ability to metabolize up to 30% of its volume, meaning the medicine could feel more powerful.[29] Having too much of <u>any</u> kind of medication in the body can lead to a host of negative issues, up to and including death, depending on potency and dosage. While the list of side effects from cannabis does not include death and might not be as severe as other prescriptions, there is still potential for cannabis to have an interaction with other medications. So, the age of the cannabis consumer is an especially important topic for those who want to take cannabis for chronic conditions. Consistent dosing is far more important for those consuming medicinally as compared to those consuming cannabis recreationally.

New Consumers of Cannabis

Absorption of Cannabis

There are so many different factors to consider when taking cannabis as a medicine, including how it is prepared, how our bodies absorb the cannabis, and the metabolism of the person taking cannabis. The way the cannabis is prepared plays a large role in whether or not the cannabis consumer will feel any of the intended effects. Cannabis is naturally fat-loving (fat-soluble) and water-hating (water-insoluble). This means that it will more readily bind to foods that are higher in fat, like milk, butter, oils, peanut butter, etc. If a person consumed cannabis without adding any type of fat into the preparation, there could potentially be a minimal or no effect on the body. But cannabis that has been infused into butter or oil (or any fat) will be easier for the body to absorb and break down.

Recently, research has brought about some amazing techniques for preparing cannabis in such a way as to make it water-soluble (water-loving).[30] These new advancements in cannabis preparation have led to the production of powders that can be mixed into drinks to make cannabis beverages. However, water-soluble forms of cannabis are more easily found within dispensaries rather than made at home. As long as you have access to a kitchen and basic cooking utensils, you can infuse cannabis into an oil or butter to consume, but few will have access to the machines that are needed to create cannabis drinks.

Cannabis Dosing Considerations

If this is your first time consuming cannabis of any sort (or even if you have consumed cannabis in the past, but it has been some time since), starting at a low dose and slowly working your way up is the most appropriate way to go.

Multiple research studies and the Cannabis Nurses Association have shown that a reasonable starting dose for cannabis is 1.25 mg – 2.5 mg per day in adults if you are taking an oral (pill or food) preparation.[13, 14, 31] Finding the right cannabis dosage is a very individual process, and some experimentation may be needed to find the most effective dosage for your symptoms. One of the reasons that finding the right cannabis dosage can be such a process is due to the fact that it's not entirely dependent on a person's height, size, or weight; it is dependent on the individual person's endocannabinoid system (ECS).

Whenever cannabis is eaten, it has the potential to last within the body and produce an effect anywhere from 4 to 12 hours after consumption.[14] For this reason, it is better to start low and increase the dosage of cannabis slowly over 3-4 days.[14] A good rule of thumb is to not increase the cannabis dosage by more than your current dosage of cannabis. For example, say your starting dose was 1.25 mg, and you gave it 3 to 4 days to see what effect it had upon your symptoms, but it didn't give the desired effect, you would want to increase your dosage by another 1.25 mg.[14] Increasing by more than the previous dose could also increase the chances of experiencing negative side effects as the total dosage goes up.[14] Just be aware that doubling your dose at, say, 5 or 10 mg is not the same as doubling your dose at 50 or 100 mg. In fact, I would highly encourage extreme caution when doubling up the cannabis dosage as you get close to or over 25 mg. Besides the increased chance of side effects, you will want to consider the financial impact – a higher dose comes at a higher price. To summarize, increasing your dosage slowly is the preferred method.

We have briefly discussed the various aspects that can affect how quickly or slowly cannabis can be absorbed within the body when taking cannabis via the oral route, but a person's metabolism also impacts the absorption of medicines. A person who is young and healthy might have a higher metabolism, which can increase the rate at which edibles are broken down in the body, whereas a person who is older or someone who has liver issues might be slower to metabolize cannabis and therefore feel the effects of cannabis more and potentially longer. An important note: if you have been diagnosed with something that affects your liver, it is incredibly important to talk with the doctor who manages your liver symptoms before starting cannabis. Cannabis is metabolized by the liver and could cause more harm than benefit if it is not filtered out of the body properly. The digestive tract also has a part to play in the metabolism of cannabis. If food moves slowly through the digestive tract, it could take longer for a person to feel the effects of cannabis. Whereas if food is moving through the digestive tract quickly, it will make it to the stomach quicker to be broken down.

Introduction to Cannabinoids, Flavonoids, and Terpenes

In this section, we will cover the different classes of compounds that can be found in the cannabis plant. Each section will start with a summary of what we currently know about the different compound classes, followed by a brief look at the individual compounds within each class and what they could do for us. As previously mentioned, research into the cannabis plant is still in its infancy, so the potential that we'll eventually learn of more compounds than those listed here is quite high. However, learning and understanding the differences between cannabinoids, flavonoids, and terpenes, especially in how each of these compounds could benefit us, is incredibly important to make an informed selection of medications. If, for example, we as consumers know that cultivars with higher amounts of CBG alleviate our chronic pain and inflammation, then we are less likely to pick a cultivar that is lacking CBG when visiting the dispensary.

In the upcoming sections you will see the chemical formula for the different components of cannabis right beside the name of the compound. These are placed here as a visual reminder that these are in fact chemical compounds that can be synthesized, like Epidiolex, which is prescribed for severe seizures. Cannabis can be altered in a lab quite easily as well, such as with Δ8-THC. I also found it quite interesting to see the differences and similarities between the compounds.

Cannabinoids

Cannabinoids are a class of chemical compounds that act on the endocannabinoid receptors in our brains and elsewhere in the body. They also support the physiologic functions of the endocannabinoid system (ECS), meaning they help support the ECS as it works.[14] There are endocannabinoids (endo = within) that our bodies make, such as anandamide, and there are exogenous (exo = from without) phytocannabinoids that come from various plant sources, such as THC and CBD that come from cannabis.[14] Some of the most commonly recognized cannabinoids are THC and CBD as they are the most abundant within cannabis, but there are over 120 (!) different cannabinoids that have been discovered.[32] Some of the most abundant cannabinoids found in cannabis include Δ-9-THC, Δ-8-THC, CBD, CBN, CBG, CBC, THCV, CBV and CBDV.[33] Other cannabinoids can be found within cannabis, but generally in lower quantities. The following section describes the specific cannabinoids within the cannabis plant and what we currently know about them.

THC – Tetrahydrocannabinol

THC is easily the most recognizable cannabinoid from the cannabis plant. It is the only compound that causes the psychoactive and intoxicating aspect that some people pursue. THC has been shown to help maintain a normal inflammatory response, support sleep, and combat nausea.[14] The current research has shown that THC demonstrates a myriad of positive effects, such as:

- Helps maintain the normal moisture content of the skin. Dry skin occurs when the skin doesn't retain

sufficient moisture either as a result of frequent bathing, use of harsh soaps, cold/dry air, aging, as well as certain medical conditions.[34] Cannabis helps the skin retain moisture by supporting the body's natural processes.
- Helps relieve occasional joint stiffness.
- Offers antioxidant protection.
- Helps maintain a normal inflammatory response.
- May provide a calming effect on nerves in small doses.
- Supports normal respiratory function in small doses.
- May support normal neurological function.

Research has shown that smaller amounts of THC can be incredibly effective at reducing symptoms, while larger doses of THC may actually intensify symptoms such as an increased heart rate and anxiety.[14] When first trying out THC, it is best practice to start at a small dose, as we discussed in the section about Dosing Considerations. According to the Journal of Cannabis Research, the maximum daily dose of THC is 40 mg/day or less depending on the condition[13] however, research is consistently being released on this subject.

CBD – Cannabidiol

The second most readily identifiable cannabinoid is cannabidiol or CBD. This compound of the cannabis plant has increased in popularity seemingly overnight but, in reality, has been consumed for quite some time. CBD was recently removed from Schedule I status (see Definition List) due to the 2018 Farm Bill that defined hemp as having less than 0.3% THC total dry weight.[8] While hemp plants have less than 0.3% THC, those same plants tend to have far more of the non-psychoactive compounds like CBD. So far, clinical trials (both pre-clinical and in process) have demonstrated that CBD has the following effects:

- Helps support normal neurological function.
- Helps maintain a normal inflammatory response.
- Promotes movement and healthy joints.
- Offers antioxidant protection.
- Has calming effects on the nerves.
- Helps maintain a normal emotional balance.
- Supports normal neurological function.[15]

CBN – Cannabinol

CBN is not as well-known as CBD or THC but has seen an increase in popularity recently and is predominately known for its help in maintaining a healthy sleep routine. CBN is unique in that this compound is formed as THC is exposed to light, heat, and with the passage of time.[35] CBN is naturally created in one of three ways. 1) Naturally, by waiting to harvest the cannabis flowers until the trichomes (see Definitions List) have turned an amber or gold color. 2) By exposure to heat or light. This is especially important to know as some dispensaries will display and dispense their flower in glass jars. 3) The last way that THC degrades to CBN is by the passing of time, even if the cannabis flower is stored well (kept in a cool, dark place). Researchers have found that an average of 11.8% THC will degrade to CBN over 30 days' time, and 34.6% will degrade down over 360 days. Current research has shown that CBN demonstrates the following properties:[35]

- May have a calming effect on the nerves.
- Helps maintain normal neurologic function.
- Assists in maintaining a normal inflammatory response.
- May support the proper balance of normal intestinal flora.
- May have some activity against MRSA (Methicillin-resistant *Staphylococcus aureus*).[15]

The amount of CBN in the plant can be directly related to how cannabis is stored and the passage of time, as studies have shown that 41% of THC converts to CBN after four years have passed.[35]

CBG – Cannabigerol

CBG is another compound of the cannabis plant that is being researched more and more recently. This cannabinoid is not often found in cultivars that are high in THC. CBG has received the nickname the "mother of all cannabinoids" due to the way different compounds are created in the cannabis plant. Inside the cannabis plant, this compound starts out as CBGA, which is then converted into almost all other cannabinoids through photosynthesis as the plant grows (CBGA → CBG → almost all other cannabinoids).[31] This is an incredibly interesting compound and has a variety of exciting possible uses. Research shows that CBG has the following characteristics:

- CBG is non-psychoactive; it will not make you high.
- May help support normal neurologic function.

- May support the proper balance of normal intestinal flora.[15]
- May have some activity against MRSA (Methicillin-resistant *Staphylococcus aureus*).[15]
- May help more GABA (see definition) transmitters be available for use within the body. This could potentially help with a variety of issues, such as seizures, convulsions, anxiety, insomnia, muscle tremors, and analgesics.
- May help to maintain normal immune function.

CBC – Cannabichromene

CBC is one of the more abundant cannabinoids after THC and CBD but still occurs in relatively low amounts in most cultivars.[15] Throughout history, CBC was one of the most abundant phytocannabinoids (see Definitions List) in the cannabis plant. But in recent years, growers of cannabis have hybridized the plant so many different times/ways, looking to get the highest CBD and THC levels, which in turn has decreased the amount of CBC found in cannabis plants.[37] CBC has been shown to help support normal inflammatory response (in fact helping the human body do what it is supposed to do) and to help boost the effects of THC.[15] CBC is also being researched to determine its role in the fields of cancer, pain, and inflammation.[14] CBC has been known to demonstrate the following properties:

- May help reduce inflammation-induced hypermotility in the gut. This could potentially be helpful in irritable bowel-type situations.
- Is not psychoactive, i.e. will not make you high.

- May have anti-nociceptive (anti-pain) effects. Anti-nociceptive refers to how CBC could help block the detection of a painful or injurious stimulus by our sensory neurons. To break this down a bit further, CBC tells your pain receptors not to feel pain.[38, 39]

THCV – Tetrahydrocannabivarin

THCV is a slightly more unique cannabinoid in that it does not originate from CBGA, one of the growth pathways for cannabis compounds. Instead, THCV originates from the precursor cannabigeroveric acid (CBGVA) and then is converted to THCV. Because of its unique structure, THCV can have a protective effect (at low doses) against the negative side effects of THC, but at higher doses, it may increase the negative side effects of THC. THCV may help support a healthy weight, normal endocrine function, normal neurological function, and normal muscle movements.[14] THCV has been shown to have the following properties:

- THCV can have appetite-suppressant properties.[40]
- Has some interesting possibilities when it comes to controlling blood sugars in people with diabetes.[40]
- Low doses of THCV may help reduce the side effects brought on by THC.[14]
- Potential anti-seizure effect by supporting normal neurological function.[15]

CBDV – Cannabidivarin

CBDV is a relatively new on the cannabinoid in the cannabis world, and while research is still limited, early studies suggest it may support normal neurological functions, particularly in cases of partial-onset seizures.[15] Additionally, it has been linked to promoting normal gastric emptying. Unlike THC, CBDV is non-psychoactive, meaning it doesn't produce a "high." It has shown promising results in treating difficult-to-manage seizure disorders, such as drug-resistant epilepsy, especially in women with Rett Syndrome.[41]

This is what we currently know about CBDV:
- Research is being done to determine the role of CBDV in nerve inflamation.[42]
- Research into CBDV and its relationship with autism is being done.[43]
- CBDV is structurally similar to CBD, and so has similar properties.[41]
- Has possible health benefits for people dealing with seizures and increased gastric motility.[41]

CBV - Cannabivarin

CBV is a cannabinoid that truly has very little research completed on it as of the date of this publication. Currently, CBV is being studied to see how (or if) it has an effect on weight loss, insomnia, and cancer.[44]

The properties of CBV as we know it are:
- Not psychoactive; it will not get you high.
- May act on the body similarly to THC.[44]

Terpenes

Terpenes may be an entirely new concept to some, but it is one of the largest and most diverse groups of naturally occurring compounds in both cannabis and other plants.[45] Terpenes were originally discovered as a separate category from cannabinoids by researchers named Simonsen and Todd in 1942 who identified that terpenes were present in all plants.[46] Terpenes are aromatic oils that are secreted from the same cannabis oil glands (trichomes) that produce cannabinoids. They are responsible for the various fragrances and flavors of cannabis and may influence cannabis' effects. Terpenes have a variety of characteristics, including flavor, smell, effects, and medicinal potential. The six most prevalent fragrances and flavors are clove, lemon, pine, floral, pepper, and fragrant wood.[14]

As cannabis has become more popular as a medicine and a method of relaxation, terpenes have also recently come into the spotlight, and we have learned that there are over 50,000 terpenes found in nature, 100 of which are specific to cannabis.[14] Terpenes can be classified in several different ways, most often based on the location of a certain molecule (C_5H_8, an isoprene molecule) on the chemical structure.[14] Continue reading to learn more about the various individual terpenes that are commonly found in the cannabis plant.

Myrcene

Aroma: earthy, musky, and resembling cloves.

The reported effects of myrcene are:

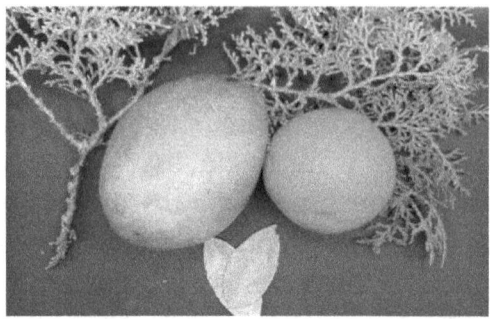

Photo 10 - Cypress, mango, bay leaves, citrus fruit

- May promote a normal pain response.
- Helps support a normal inflammation response.
- May help protect body cells and tissues.
- Supports the proper balance of normal intestinal flora.
- May offer antioxidant protection.
- May help support normal brain function and
- Supports normal sleep and relaxation.

Myrcene is also found in bay leaves, pine, juniper, citrus fruit, hops, eucalyptus, mango, and thyme. It is abundantly found in hops and is the most prevalent terpene found in cannabis. Interestingly enough, myrcene is also used as the starting material for commercially important scents and flavors such as menthol, nerol, geraniol, and linalool.[14, 14, 47]

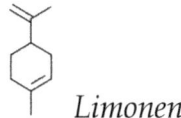 *Limonene*

Aroma: lemon, lime, and orange.

The reported effects of limonene are:

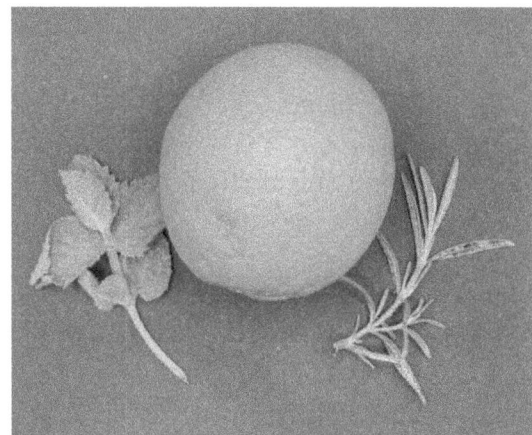

Photo 11 - Mint, citrus and rosemary

- May support antioxidant protection.
- Has a calming effect on nerves.
- May help protect body cells and tissues.
- May support the proper balance of normal intestinal flora.
- May help support overall gut health.

Limonene is also found in citrus rind, pine, mint, rosemary and juniper. It is the second most abundant monoterpene (see Definitions List) found in cannabis. An interesting fact about limonene is that it is a major component of citrus essential oil and is widely used as a flavoring agent in foods, cosmetics, medical products, personal care items and cleaning products.[14, 15, 48]

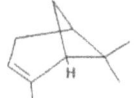 *Pinene*

Aroma: pine and fir tree-like.

The reported effects of pinene are:

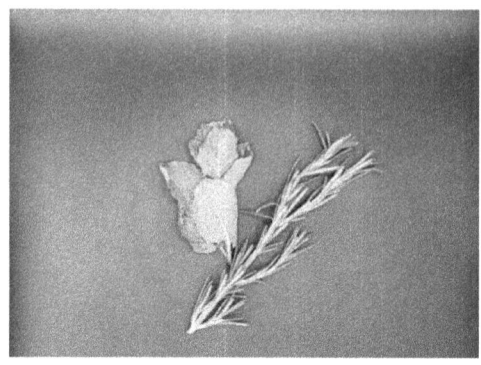
Photo 12 - Mint and rosemary

- May help support a normal inflammation response.
- May help support normal respiratory functions.
- May help support normal mucus function.
- May help protect body cells and tissues.
- May support normal pain function.
- May support normal neurological function.

Pinene is also found in pine trees, balsamic resin, rosemary, basil and eucalyptus. It is also a monoterpene and is one of the most abundant terpenes existing in nature. Pinene has a 60% bioavailability through the inhalation route, meaning it works really well when inhaled. This terpene is also attributed to the success of "shinrin-yoku" or "forest bathing" which is practiced in Japan and involves taking in the forest atmosphere to feel relaxed.[14, 15, 49, 50]

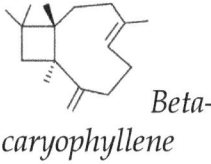 *Beta-caryophyllene*

Aroma: a peppery, fragrant wood and spicy scent.

The reported effects of beta-caryophyllene are:

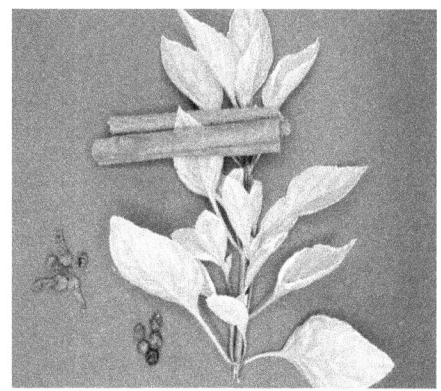

Photo 13 - Cloves, black pepper, cinnamon and basil

- May help support a normal inflammation response.
- Has a calming effect on nerves.
- May help protect body cells and tissues.
- Supports a normal pain function.

Beta-caryophyllene is also found in cedarwood, black pepper, rosemary, cloves, basil, oregano, lavender, cinnamon and hops. This terpene is the most common sesquiterpene (see Definition List) and is the only terpene that binds directly, although weakly, to the CB2 receptor, making it both a cannabinoid and a terpenoid.[14] Interestingly enough, caryophyllene is the primary scent that police dogs are trained to detect and is often associated with cultivars high in THC.[14] This terpene plays a major role in copaiba oil, which is an important anti-inflammatory herbal medicine of the Brazilian Amazon.[15]

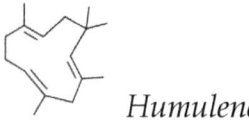 *Humulene*

Aroma: earthy, fragrant wood and spicy.

The reported effects of humulene are:

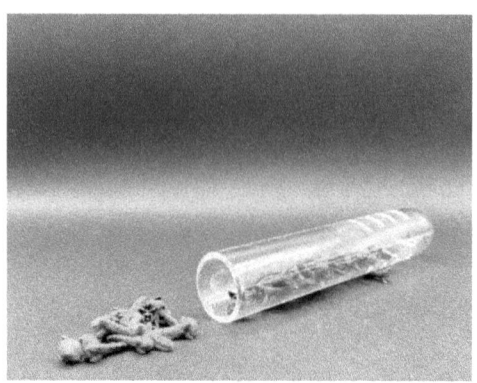
Photo 14 - Cloves

- May help support normal eating patterns.
- May help support a normal inflammation response.
- May help protect body cells and tissues.
- May help support a normal pain function.

Humulene is also found in clove, sage, ginseng, black pepper and hops. It is also known as alpha-caryophyllene as it shares the same chemical formula as beta-caryophyllene but differs in the structure. Humulene is abundantly found in the hops plant.[14, 15, 51]

Linalool

Aroma: lavender with a hint of spice.

The reported effects of linalool are:

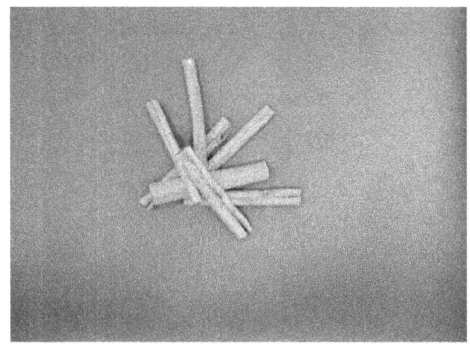

Photo 15 - Cinnamon

- May help support a normal inflammation response.
- May help calm nerves.
- Supports a normal neurological response.

Linalool is also found in cinnamon, coriander, lavender, mint, rosewood and birch trees. It has been researched rather often for its anxiolytic (anti-anxiety) effects, but little is yet known about the underlying mechanism. When researched in mice, linalool seems to have the best effect on anxiety when it is smelled (such as is the case with smelling lavender).[14, 15, 52]

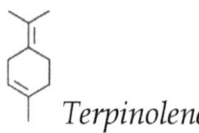 *Terpinolene*

Aroma: piney and herbal with floral hints.

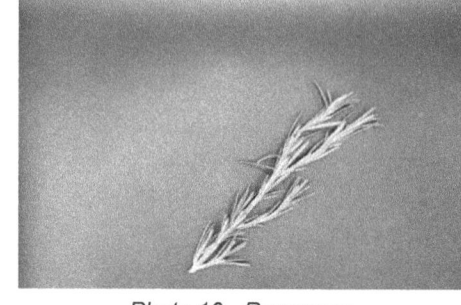
Photo 16 - Rosemary

The reported effects of terpinolene are that it has a calming effect on the nerves and helps support normal neurological function.[14]

Terpinolene is also found in allspice, juniper, parsnips, pine, rosemary, sage and tea tree. The presence of terpinolene within cannabis is said to be characteristic of "sativa" (referring to the uplifting/energizing feeling) varieties. Some studies have shown that terpinolene has sedative effects in mice, but in humans it has been noted that terpinolene has stimulating effects.[14, 15]

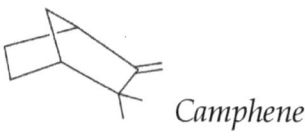 *Camphene*

Aroma: damp woodlands, fir needles and musky earth.

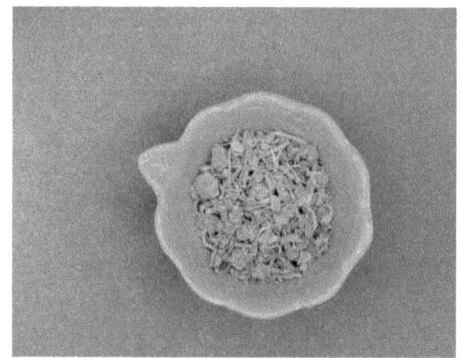
Photo 17 - Valerian root

The reported effect of camphene is that it helps support a normal cholesterol function.

Camphene is also found in conifers, nutmeg, cypress, bergamot and valerian. It is most notably found in camphor oil which has been commonly used in Asia for centuries. Camphor was one of the strong fragrances used during the times of the Black Death in 14th century Europe to reduce the smell of rotting corpses.[14, 53]

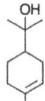 *Terpineol*

Aroma: lilacs and apple blossom with a hint of citrus.

The reported effects of terpineol are:

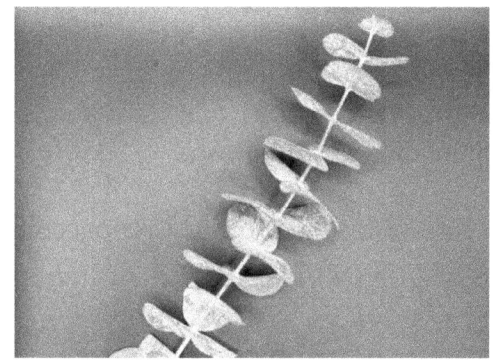
Photo 18 - Eucalyptus

- May help protect body cells and tissues.
- May help support antioxidant protection.
- Has a calming effect on the nerves.

Terpineol is also found in pine trees, balsamic resin, rosemary, basil and eucalyptus. This terpene can occur in four different chemical structures but is most commonly found as alpha-terpineol. Terpineol is often used in soap or lotion recipes because of its pleasant aroma.[14, 54]

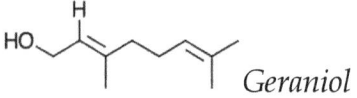 *Geraniol*

Aroma: floral and occasionally fruity.

The reported effects of geraniol are that it may offer antioxidant protection and helps to support "normal" neurological function.

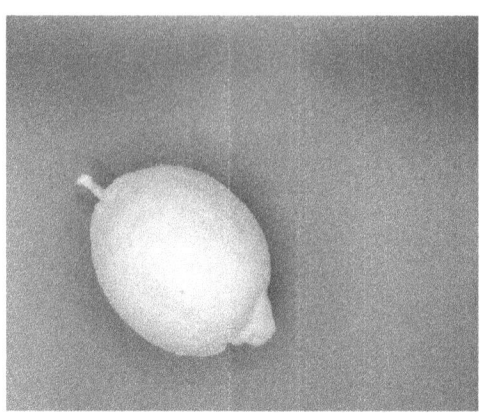

Photo 19 - Lemons

Geraniol is also found in tobacco and lemon and is known to repel mosquitos.[14, 54]

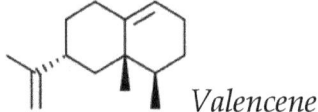 *Valencene*

Aroma: citrusy, reminiscent of oranges, grapefruits and occasionally of fresh herbs or freshly cut wood.

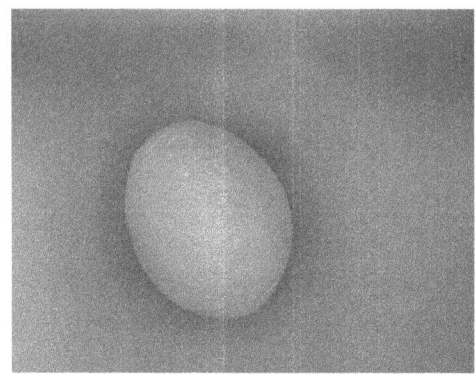

Photo 20 - Oranges

The reported effect of valencene is that it may help support a normal inflammation response.

This terpene is also found in Valencia oranges and is commonly used as an insect and tick repellent.[14, 54]

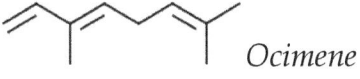 *Ocimene*

Aroma: sweet, fragrant, herbaceous and woodsy.

The reported effects of ocimene are:

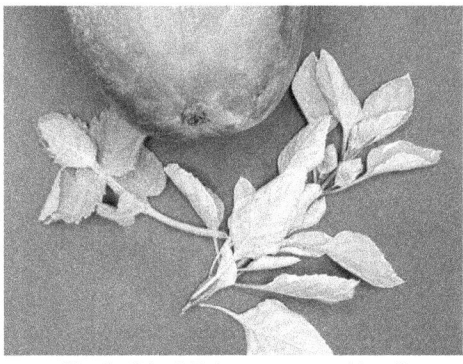

Photo 21 - Mint, mango and basil

- May help support a normal inflammation response.
- May help support normal viral function.
- Supports the proper balance of normal intestinal flora.

Ocimene is also found in mint, mangoes, basil and orchids. Little research has been done even in other plants besides cannabis, but this terpene is commonly used as a fragrance for everyday items like perfume and deodorant.[14, 55]

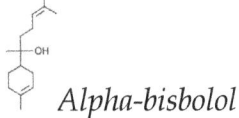 *Alpha-bisbolol*

Aroma: light, sweet and floral.

The reported effects of alpha-bisbolol are that it

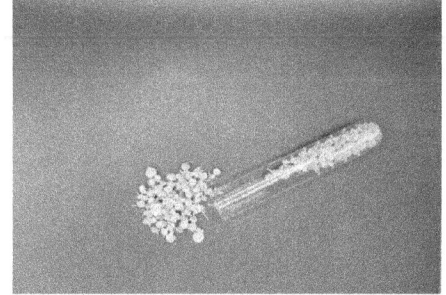

Photo 22 - Chamomile

may help protect body cells and tissues, as well as may support a normal pain function.

Alpha-bisbolol is also found in chamomile flowers and candeia trees (found in South America). It is commonly used in teas, makeup, shampoos and lotions as a fragrance.[14, 55]

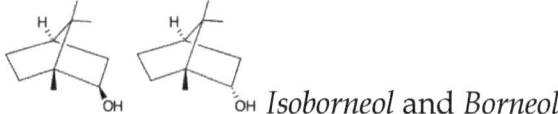 *Isoborneol* and *Borneol*

Aroma: strong, bitter aroma.

The reported effects of isoborneol and borneol are that it is used as an insect repellent and may help protect body cells and tissues.

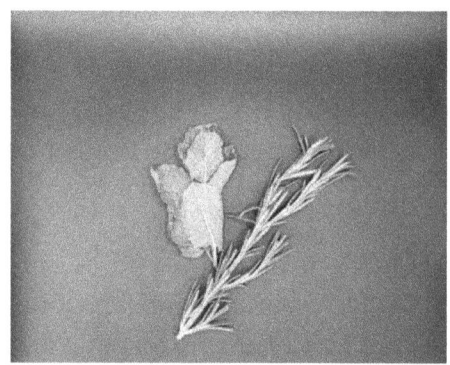
Photo 23 - Mint and rosemary

Isoborneol and borneol are also found in rosemary, mint and camphor. They are most often used in baked goods due to their flavor and are a staple in traditional Chinese medicine.[14, 55]

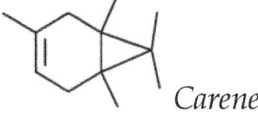
Carene

Aroma: pungent and sweet citrus.

The reported effects of carene are:

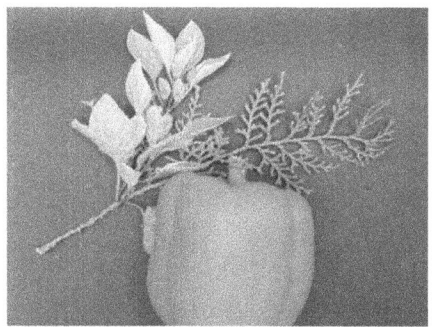
Photo 24 - Basil, bell pepper and cedar

- May alleviate pain.
- May support neurological function.
- Supports the inflammatory function.

Carene is also found in rosemary, basil, bell peppers, cedar and pine. It is largely used in cosmetics and perfumes. Caution must be exercised with this terpene as overexposure to carene can cause irritation to the skin, eyes and lungs.[14, 56, 57]

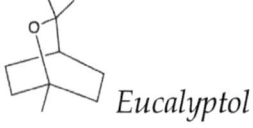 *Eucalyptol*

Aroma: fresh, minty aroma and cooling taste.

The reported effects of eucalyptol are:

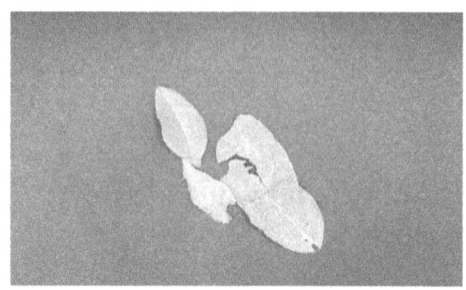

Photo 25 - Bay leaves

- May help support normal pain response.
- May help protect body cells and tissues.
- Supports the balance of normal intestinal flora.

Eucalyptol is also found in eucalyptus, sweet basil, bay leaves, camphor laurel trees and tea trees. Prior to standardized medicines, eucalyptol was often used as a cough suppressant.[14, 55]

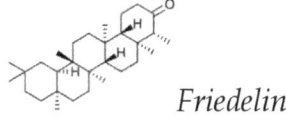 *Eudesmol*

Aroma: woody and refreshing.

The reported effects of eudesmol are:

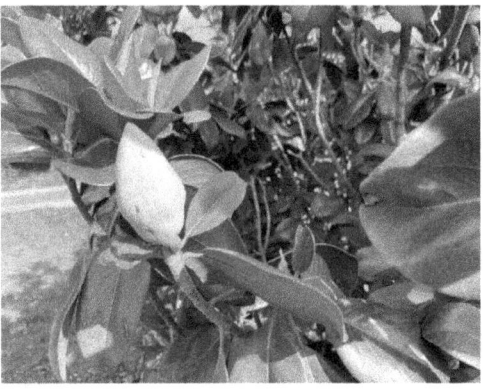
Photo 26 - Magnolia Tree

- May help support a normal inflammation response.
- Supports the normal neurological function.

Eudesmol is also found in magnolia trees and ginkgo biloba. Currently researchers are studying eudesmol and how it stimulates gastric emptying as well as intestinal motility.[58]

Friedelin

Aroma: odorless.

The reported effects of friedelin are:

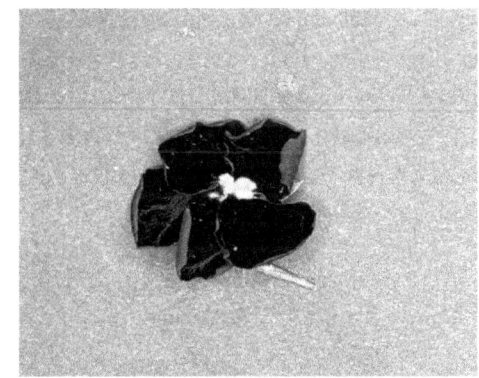
Photo 27 - Violets

- May help support a normal inflammation response.
- May help support a normal fever response.
- May help protect body cells and tissues.

Friedelin is also found in rhododendron, algae, lichen, violets, mosses and peat. It is the most prevalent triterpenoid (see Definitions List) found in cannabis and is specifically found in the roots of the cannabis plant.[15, 59]

Guaiol

Aroma: floral.

The reported effects of guaiol are:

- May help protect body cells and tissues.
- May offer antioxidant protection.

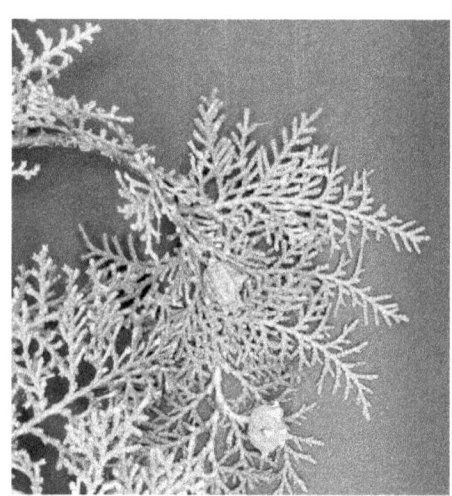

Photo 28 - Cypress

Guaiol is also found in guaiacum, pine and cypress. Interestingly, guaiol has been found to be used by many cultures as early as the 16th Century.[14, 55]

cis-Nerolidol

Aroma: freshly cut wood and fruity aroma.

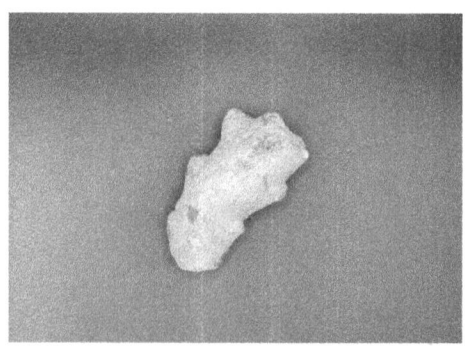

Photo 29 - Ginger

The reported effects of cis-nerolidol are:

- May help support a normal inflammation response.
- May offer antioxidant support.

cis-Nerolidol is also found in jasmine, ginger, honeysuckle and lavender. There are two different chemical structures associated with Nerolidol. cis-Nerolidol is the most prevalent terpene in the cannabis plant.[14, 55]

trans-Nerolidol

Aroma: woody, fruity and citrus aroma.

The reported effects of trans-Nerolidol are:

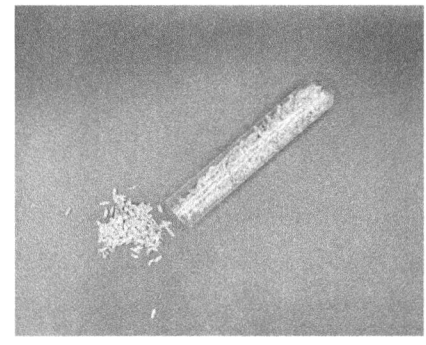
Photo 30 - Lavender

- Helps support proper balance of normal intestinal flora.
- Offers antioxidant protection.

trans-Nerolidol is also found in jasmine, lavender, lemongrass and tea tree oil. It is commonly used in lotions and perfumes for its scent as well as in candy and chewing gum for its flavor.[14, 55]

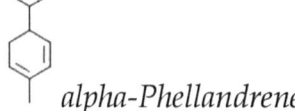 *alpha-Phellandrene*

Aroma: peppery.

The reported effects of alpha-phellandrene are:

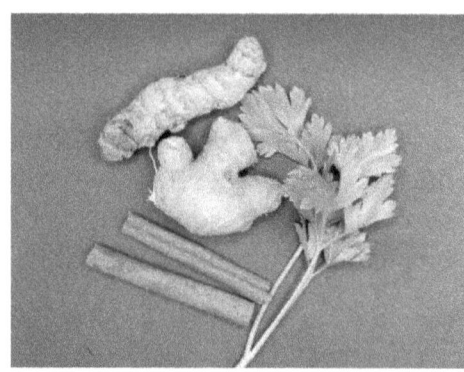

Photo 31 - Turmeric, ginger, cinnamon and parsley

- May help protect body cells and tissues.
- Supports the proper balance of normal intestinal flora.

alpha-Phellandrene is also found in cinnamon, garlic, dill, ginger, parsley, turmeric and eucalyptus oil. It is commonly used as a fragrance as well as a food additive.[14, 55]

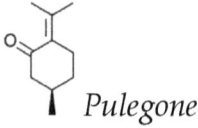 *Pulegone*

Aroma: mint-like.

The reported effects of pulegone are:

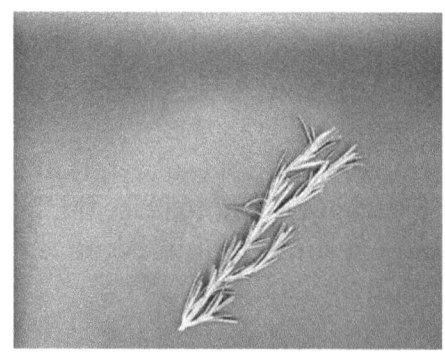

Photo 32 - Rosemary

- Has a calming effect on the nerves.
- Helps support a normal fever function.

Pulegone is also found in rosemary and is commonly used in cosmetics, food and perfumes.[14, 60, 61]

Sabinene

Aroma: spicy scent and flavor.

The reported effects of Sabinene are:

- Offers antioxidant protection.
- Helps support a normal inflammation response.

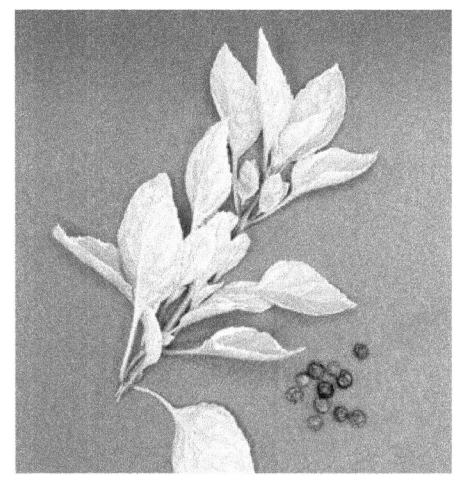
Photo 33 - Basil and black pepper

Sabinene is also found in black pepper and basil. It is not as commonly found in large amounts within the cannabis plant.[14, 57] Cannabis cultivars that are higher in sabinene are from the Haze family, such as Super Silver Haze.[62]

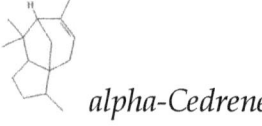 *alpha-Cedrene*

Aroma: fresh, woody, and sweet scent.

The reported effects of alpha-Cedrene are:

- Helps support normal immune function.
- May help protect body cells and tissues.

Photo 34 – Cedar tree

alpha-Cedrene is also found in cedar, juniper and cypress wood. It is not found in abundance within cannabis but is there. It is most commonly used in soaps, candles, cleaning agents, and insect repellents.[55, 63]

Farnesene

Aroma: fruity, like green apples.

The reported effects of farnesene are:

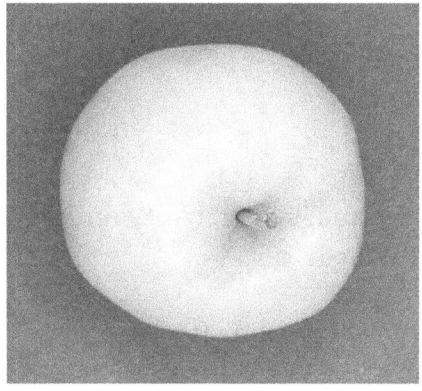
Photo 35 - Green apples

- Helps support a normal inflammation response.
- Supports the proper balance of normal intestinal function.
- Helps calm nerves.

Farnesene is also found in green apples. It is one of the less commonly found terpenes in cannabis but can be found in cultivars such as Gainsville Green and Cherry Punch.[64]

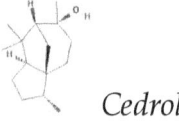 *Cedrol*

Aroma: sweet, fruity and cedar-like.

The reported effects of cedrol are:

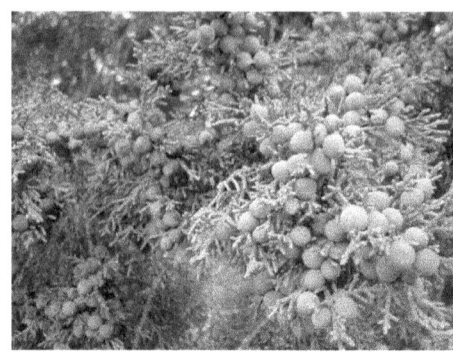

Photo 36 - Juniper

- May help protect body cells and tissues.
- Supports the proper balance of normal intestinal flora.

Cedrol is also found in cedar, cypress, juniper and oregano and is commonly used as an insect repellent.[55, 65]

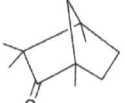 *Fenchone*

Aroma: robust, woodsy scent.

The reported effects of fenchone are:

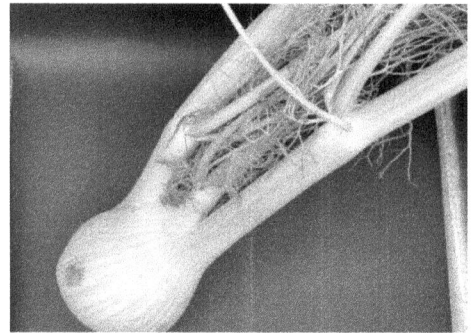

Photo 37 - Fennel

- Helps support a normal inflammation response.
- Offers antioxidant protection.
- Supports the proper balance of normal flora.

Fenchone is also found in fennel, Spanish lavender, the thuja tree and cedarwood. This terpene serves as a flavour and aroma enhancer in cannabis.[55]

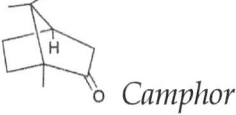
Geranyl acetate

Aroma: floral and fruity scent.

The reported effects of geranyl acetate are:

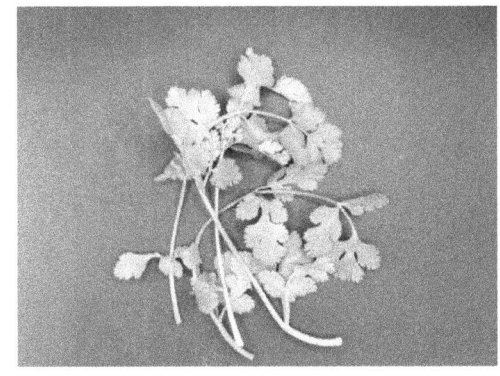
Photo 38 - Coriander (Cilantro)

- May help protect body cells and tissues.
- Supports the proper balance of normal intestinal flora.
- Helps support normal pain response.

Geranyl acetate is also found in lemongrass, coriander, sassafras, celery, almond seeds and coffee. This terpene has historically been used for many years in traditional Chinese medicine.[55]

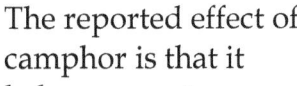 *Camphor*

Aroma: woodsy scent.

The reported effect of camphor is that it helps support a normal inflammation response.

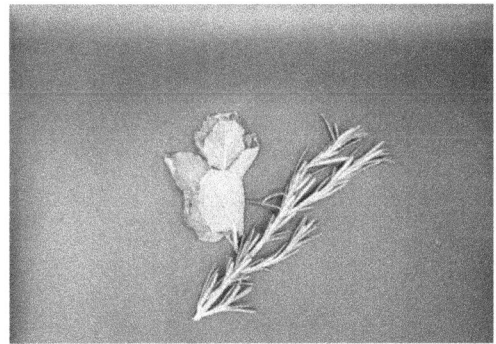
Photo 39 - Rosemary and mint

Camphor is also found in the camphor laurel tree, the Kapur tree, rosemary leaves and in the mint family. This terpene is commonly used as a fragrance additive for lotions and ointments.[55]

Nerol

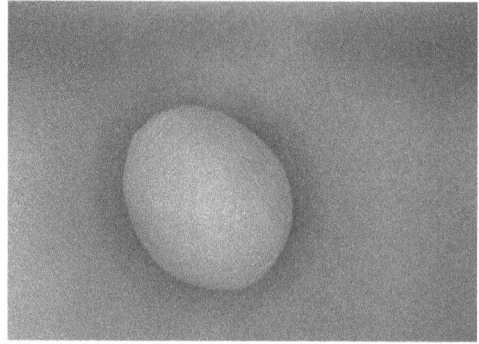

Photo 40 - Bitter oranges

Aroma: citrus and rose scent.

The reported effects of nerol are:

- Helps support a normal inflammation response.
- Helps support the proper balance of normal intestinal flora.

Nerol is also found in bitter orange trees. Interestingly enough, this terpene is a popular food additive that creates popular flavour profiles, like raspberry and red apple.[55]

Terpinene

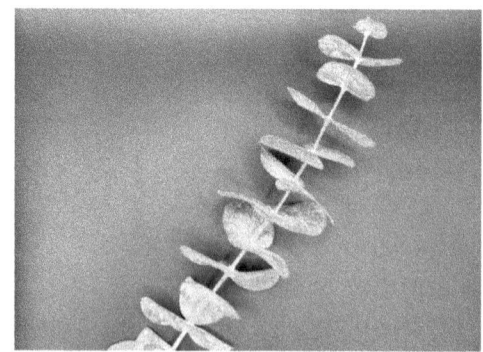

Photo 18 - Eucalyptus

Aroma: citrus-like, a spicy scent.

The reported effects of terpinene are:

- Offers antioxidant properties.
- Supports the proper balance of normal intestinal flora.

Terpinene is also found in cardamom, marjoram, juniper, and eucalyptus. This terpene has three different chemical structures known as monoterpenes and is a commonly used flavouring agent.[55] We see one of the chemical structures, alpha-pinene most often in cannabis.[14]

Flavonoids

We've learned a lot about the different compounds in the cannabis plant so far and now we come to the last category: flavonoids. The Journal of Nutritional Science states that flavonoids are a group of natural substances with variable structures (all the structures are ring-like in shape) and are found in fruits, vegetables, grains, bark, roots, stems, flowers, tea and wine.[66] Flavonoids have a certain effect when consumed in our daily diet, but they also provide protection to the plants they come from. Plants develop these flavonoids to help protect against UV rays and to ward off predators, fungi, and bacteria.[66] Research on these compounds is just beginning to focus on their individual properties. The current body of research on flavonoids remains limited for a few reasons. Historically, studies have concentrated on plants as a whole rather than isolating specific compounds. Additionally, many of these compounds have only recently been discovered, and research into their effects is just now starting to take shape.

It must be noted that flavonoids are not specific to the cannabis plant, they are also found in a wide variety of plants, fruits and vegetables that are easily accessed and eaten by most people. Some flavonoids lend the plant their unique color while others lend the plant the flavor that it is known for.[66] These compounds can have a profound effect on humans, pets, and the plants themselves. Future research into cannabis medicine promises to unlock a wealth of exciting, groundbreaking discoveries, opening up new possibilities and revolutionizing our understanding of this powerful plant!

While flavonoids are not often talked about when it comes to the cannabis plant, they play an emerging and important role therein. Flavonoids are important in plants as they are not only responsible for the color and aroma of plants, but they also help to attract pollinators, protect from UV light and they act as antimicrobial agents.[14] In humans, flavonoids are also known to help maintain a normal inflammatory response, offer antioxidant protection, and they have immune-enhancing effects in vitro as they modulate key cellular enzymatic functions within the body.[14] Let's consider the individual flavonoids and what they could potentially help with.

Cannflavin A and B

Cannflavin A and B are unique in that they are only found in the cannabis plant and are responsible for a variety of essential functions including protection against UV rays and warding off predators, fungi, and bacteria.[67]

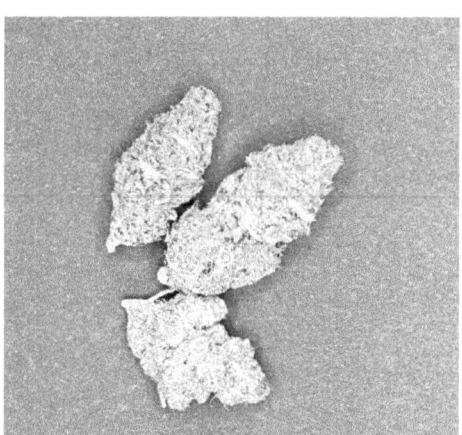

Photo 42 -Cannabis

Cannflavin A and B are yet two more compounds in the cannabis plant that are in desperate need of more research. Currently though, they are being researched to discover their role regarding antioxidant protection, regulating cellular activity and pain and inflammation reduction.[46]

Kaempferol

Kaempferol is most known for its research studies into antioxidant activity, inflammation, as well as the activity of cancer cells when they come in contact with this flavonoid.[63]

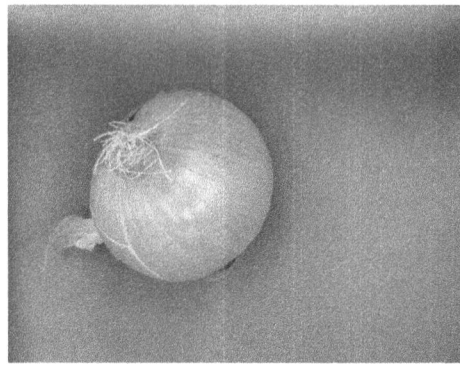

Photo 43 - Onion

This flavonoid can be found in other foods as well as cannabis, such as kale, broccoli, onions, green beans, and ginger. Kaempferol is found abundantly in green leafy vegetables that are already a staple in many diets.[69] Adding fresh vegetables to your meals could be an easy way to get more Kaempferol into your diet.

Quercetin

Quercetin is a flavonoid that is found in cannabis as well as fruits and vegetables, chocolate, red wine and olive oil. This flavonoid is currently being researched for its antioxidant and anti-inflammation activity.

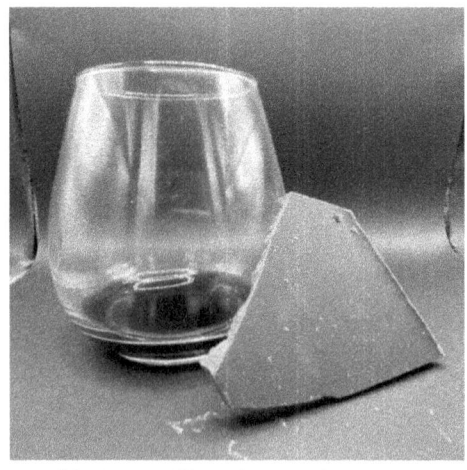

Photo 44 - Chocolate and red wine

Interestingly enough, quercetin is also prevalent in onions. The higher the quercetin amount, the more colorful the onion. Quercetin and kaempferol lend cannabis the deep purple color that some buds have. There is a lot of interesting research available on how wine and chocolate can affect a person's mood and health, some which may be due to compounds like Quercetin.[70]

Apigenin

Apigenin is a flavonoid that is naturally occurring in various fruits, vegetables and herbs, including cannabis, oranges, celery, onions, chamomile and basil.[71] This flavonoid is being researched to determine its role in clearing up skin of acne, pain relief, cancer and Alzheimer's disease.[71, 72] Apigenin is available in various fruits, vegetables and herbs, and as such could easily be added to the average daily diet.

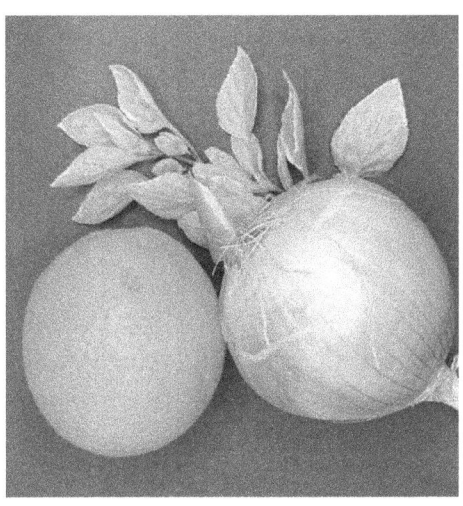

Photo 45 - Oranges, basil and onions

Chrysin

The flavonoid Chrysin is well known for its presence in flowers, such as the passion flower and silver linden tree, as well as in honey, bee propolis, and cannabis.[73] Chrysin is being researched to determine its anti-inflammatory, antineoplastic (blocking the formation of neoplasms [growths that may become cancer]),[74] antioxidant and liver protective activities.[75] Holistic medicine has been using chrysin, in its various forms, for inflammation, diabetes and to help support the body's natural functions over many years.[73] Chrysin can be found in medicinal plants and fruits such as bitter melon, wild Himalayan pear and the flowers of the common walnut.[76]

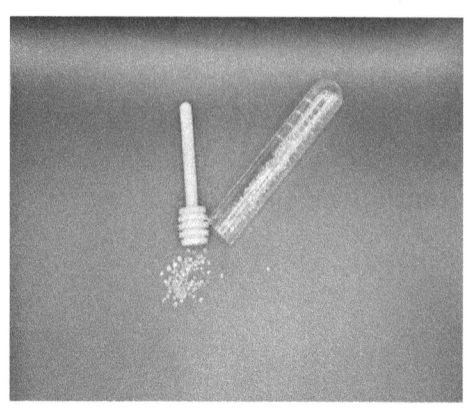

Photo 46 - Honey and bee propolis

Biacalin

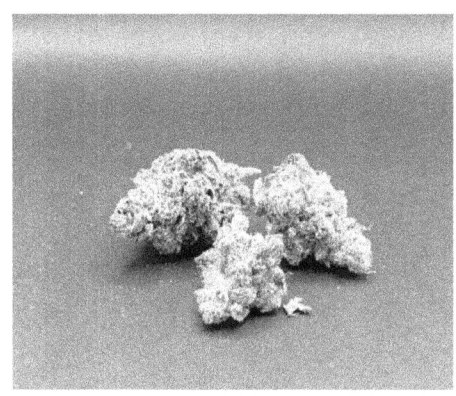
Photo 47 - Cannabis

The flavonoid biacalin is found only in small amounts within the cannabis plant but has been well studied within the Skullcap medicinal herb that is used in Chinese medicine. Skullcap is used traditionally to help support people with inflammatory diseases, tumors, diarrhea and to support longevity. Much more research still needs to be completed on how biacalin may benefit people in its isolated form, but as a part of the whole plant (the entourage effect), biacalin may help reduce inflammation and anxiety, and help support the functions of the body.[77]

Luteolin

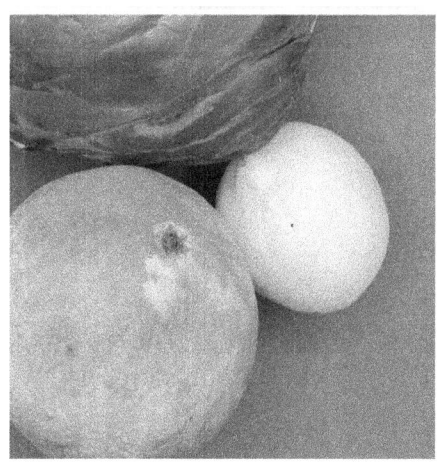
Photo 48 - Cabbage, mango and lemons

Luteolin is a well-researched flavonoid that has been called the "King of Medicines" for its multitude of uses. Luteolin is well-known as an active compound of the chebula tree that is native to Tibet, and which bears fruit that looks similar to pears. While research has not yet been fully completed to verify luteolin's effect through cannabis consumption, there is a "growing ocean of evidence for its health benefits from herbs like T. chebula." Luteolin is highest in radicchio vegetables, like purple lettuce or cabbage, as well as celery, broccoli, lemons and mangoes. [78]

Fisetin

Fisetin is another flavonoid that is present in various fruits and vegetables readily found in most grocery stores, such as strawberries, apples, grapes, onions and cucumbers.[79] This flavonoid is being researched for its potential antioxidant, neuroprotective, anti-inflammatory and longevity-supporting activities.[79] This flavonoid is incredibly interesting because of its ability to act as a senolytic, which means it breaks down old cells with damaged DNA that no longer act like normal healthy cells do.[80] The potential for flavonoids similar to Fisetin to be useful as a health supplement is quite high.

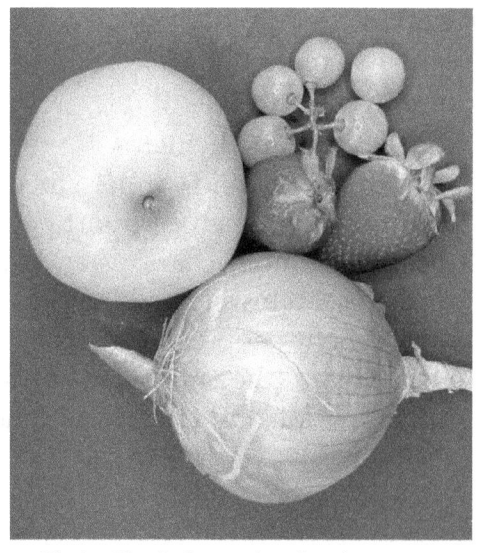

Photo 49 - Onions, strawberries, green apples and grapes

Conclusion

I hope this short booklet was able to provide you with the information you were looking for about what kinds of things you can find at an Oklahoma dispensary, the proper terminology for the cannabis plant and common definitions, as well as given a bit of insight into the time it takes for different forms of cannabis to begin taking effect in the body. The information in this booklet is but a drop in the bucket when compared to how much information and knowledge there is about cannabis to share with consumers. The cannabis plant has amazing possibilities for symptom control of aggressive disease processes, like seizures and cancer, as well as the potential to be used for less severe illnesses or symptoms. Cannabis has truly been shown to be an amazing plant!

Also in this booklet we've explored the different compounds inside the cannabis plant to gain a better understanding of how best to choose cannabis products. Having a good knowledge base of how cannabis works in the body and what the different compounds can potentially help out with, can help the medical cannabis consumer narrow down the best cultivars and products for their particular situation. With the rising prices of basically everything in our economy, being able to choose the product or cultivar that is the most effective can help keep the medicine budget under control.

While there is still so much research to be done to truly understand how cannabis works most efficiently what we do know is a positive beacon of hope for the future. I could foresee a time in the cannabis industry where once more research has been completed, cannabis consumers would be able to mix and match their favored cannabinoids, terpenes and flavonoids into tinctures or oils that could be purchased in dispensaries. Or perhaps cannabis cultivation would be so specific in the future that different cultivars could be grown for individual patients. A quick reminder that how the different compounds in cannabis work in us as medicine is called the entourage effect. In the future if we have the ability to choose specific isolated compounds as medicine, we need to also remember that the different compounds in cannabis work best in concert together (the entourage effect).[81] Whatever the future does bring in the cannabis industry, it is an actively evolving industry that I'm excited to see.

Acknowledgments

Since starting this journey of becoming a cannabis nurse educator there have been so many people supporting me through this. My sister, Cynthia Benson, helped support me emotionally through grad school when my stress and emotions were all over the place and at an all-time high. My daughter, Victory, who is an amazing teenager dealing with the grief of losing her dad, gave me strength as I continued to mourn the loss of my husband. My mom and dad, Eloisa and Charles Robinson, helped me get back on my feet after my husband died when I was in grad school and in the middle of a move. My in-laws, Dave and Cindy Shifflett, were there when I needed to talk or spend time sharing memories of Will. Another amazing person, Brandy Frisbee, was immediately excited when I told her what I wanted to do with this book and my career. Her help has been invaluable.

I would be remiss to not mention the incredible people working at Natural Remedies MMJ Dispensary in Enid. Everyone there was such a wealth of knowledge and is eager to help people learn more about cannabis; Tristan, Shea, Melissa, Mandy, Brian, and Paige are some of the names who come to mind. The Natural Remedies dispensary is my first choice when sending patients to the dispensary in Enid, OK. They care about their customers, have a wide variety of products and are always seeking different ways to educate. All of the pictures in this book that are related to cannabis products or cannabis flower come from the Natural Remedies dispensary. I cannot thank them enough for their help.

The list of people to say thank you to could be endless. There were dozens of times when a word of encouragement spoken in passing was just the thing I needed to keep moving forward. There is no way to say thank you enough. I hope you guys enjoy the book!

About the author

Christina Shifflett is a registered nurse who lives near Enid, Oklahoma, with her daughter Victory, her significant other Bram, and their silly dog, Princess Leia. Christina has had the opportunity to work in multiple disciplines in the nursing industry but has come to love educating people about cannabis the best. She graduated with a master's in Medical Cannabis Science and Therapeutics in 2022. Through this degree, she learned about the science behind cannabis as a medication, the possible interactions cannabis might have, as well as how medical cannabis can be administered.

When Christina is not providing education on cannabis, she enjoys spending time with her daughter, exploring small Oklahoma towns with Bram, and learning more about herbal medicines.

Bibliography

1. DEA. Drug Enforcement Agency on DEA website. http://tinyurl.com/4n5va9t4 10 July 2018. Accessed 18 July 2023.
2. The Science of Medicinal Cannabis (2018) *MyCannabis*. Available at: http://tinyurl.com/5fwzz57u . (Accessed: 13 June 2023).
3. Nagarkatti, P. and Nagarkatti, M. (2023) *People produce endocannabinoids – similar to compounds found in marijuana – that are critical to many bodily functions, University of South Carolina*. Available at: https://tinyurl.com/ymre29dx (Accessed: 02 April 2023).
4. Herman TF, Santos C. First Pass Effect. [Updated 2022 Jun 23]. In: *StatPearls* [Internet]. Treasure Island (FL): StatPearls Publishing; 2022 Jan-. Available from: http://tinyurl.com/bdfjfkjb (Accessed 02 April 2023).
5. What is Full Spectrum Cannabis Oil? *Care By Design*. http://tinyurl.com/yckydhhy . (Accessed 29 December 2022).
6. Cleveland Clinic medical (2022) Gamma-aminobutyric acid (GABA): What it is, Function & Benefits, Cleveland Clinic. Available at: http://tinyurl.com/45p2bmpn (Accessed: 28 July 2023).
7. Sommano SR, Chittasupho C, Ruksiriwanich W, Jantrawut P. The cannabis terpenes. *MDPI*. http://tinyurl.com/3cwsp3wt . Published December 8, 2020. (Accessed 29 December 2022).
8. Farm bill. USDA. http://tinyurl.com/5n8r6e5m . Published 2022. (Accessed 29 December 2022).
9. Physicians (2020) *Oklahoma Medical Marijuana Authority*. Available at: https://tinyurl.com/yc4j8bv3 (Accessed: 11 May 2023).

10. Medical Marijuana Act. OK. S. B. NO. 1033, entire document, 2021. http://tinyurl.com/ye255jp8 . (Accessed 29 December 2022).
11. Patient licenses (2020) *Oklahoma Medical Marijuana Authority*. Available at: https://tinyurl.com/mttw8aev (Accessed: 11 May 2022).
12. Oklahoma Medical marijuana law (2023) *NORML*. Available at: https://tinyurl.com/52k8a4j5 (Accessed: 01 May 2023).
13. Schwilke EW, Schwope DM, Karschner EL, et al. Delta9-tetrahydrocannabinol (THC), 11-hydroxy-THC, and 11-nor-9-carboxy-THC plasma pharmacokinetics during and after continuous high-dose oral THC. *Clin Chem*. 2009;55(12):2180-2189. doi:10.1373/clinchem.2008.122119. (Accessed 05 May 2023).
14. Clark CS. *Cannabis: A Handbook for Nurses*. Philadelphia: Wolters Kluwer; 2021.
15. Sulak D. *Handbook of Cannabis for Clinicians: Principles and Practice*. New York, NY, NY: W.W. Norton & Company; 2021.
16. Edible cannabis affects people differently 'start low - go slow'. (no date) *Canadian Centre on Substance Abuse and Addiction*. Available at: https://tinyurl.com/yehebjf4 (Accessed: 11 February 2023).
17. Cannabis: Inhaling vs *ingesting* (no date) *Canadian Centre on Substance Abuse and Addiction*. Available at: https://tinyurl.com/yu7jtjjv (Accessed: 11 February 2023).
18. Sublingual definition & meaning. *Merriam-Webster*. http://tinyurl.com/52ezh2yw. (Accessed 15 September 2022).
19. Buccal definition & meaning. *Merriam-Webster*. http://tinyurl.com/fuv3wznc. (Accessed 15 September 2022).

20. Buccal medicines: Giving buccal medicines. *Nationwide Children's Hospital.* http://tinyurl.com/ycyb58zu . (Accessed 15 October 2022).
21. Reeves, K.C. *et al.* (2022) 'Opioid receptor-mediated regulation of neurotransmission in the brain', *Frontiers in Molecular Neuroscience*, 15. doi:10.3389/fnmol.2022.919773.
22. Lucas P, Boyd S, Milloy MJ, Walsh Z. Cannabis Significantly Reduces the Use of Prescription Opioids and Improves Quality of Life in Authorized Patients: Results of a Large Prospective Study. *Pain Med.* 2021;22(3):727-739. doi:10.1093/pm/pnaa396
23. Marijuana. Mayo Clinic. http://tinyurl.com/4te9j5hu Published November 18, 2020. (Accessed 19 November 2022).
24. Cannabis: Overview, uses, side effects, precautions, interactions, dosing and reviews (no date) *WebMD.* Available at: http://tinyurl.com/4fce9xh6 (Accessed: 15 January 2024).
25. Niesink RJ, van Laar MW. Does Cannabidiol Protect Against Adverse Psychological Effects of THC?. Front Psychiatry. 2013;4:130. Published 2013 Oct 16. Doi:10.3389/fpsyt.2013.00130.
26. Stuyt E. The Problem with the Current High Potency THC Marijuana from the Perspective of an Addiction Psychiatrist. *Mo Med.* 2018;115(6):482-486.
27. McPartland, J.M. (1997) Cannabis as a repellant and insecticide, Cannabis as repellent and pesticide. Available at: http://tinyurl.com/mr325ze8 (Accessed: 16 January 2024).
28. D'Souza DC, Cortes-Briones JA, Ranganathan M, et al. Rapid changes in cannabinoid 1 receptor availability in cannabis-dependent male subjects after abstinence from cannabis. *Biological Psychiatry: Cognitive Neuroscience and Neuroimaging.* 2016;1(1):60-67. doi:10.1016/j.bpsc.2015.09.008

29. Drenth-van Maanen AC, Wilting I, Jansen PA. Prescribing medicines to older people — how to consider the impact of ageing on human organ and body functions. *British Journal of Clinical Pharmacology.* 2019;86(10):1921-1930. doi:10.1111/bcp.14094
30. How to get water-soluble cannabinoids for cannabis beverages (2023) *Precision Extraction Solutions.* Available at: https://tinyurl.com/yw8jjfvz (Accessed: 02 November 2023).
31. Clark PhD, RN, AHN-BC, C.S. et al (2019). Scope and standards of practice for cannabis nurses, American Cannabis Nurses Association. Available at: https://tinyurl.com/8wud6ttn . (Accessed 20 April 2024).
32. Morales P, Hurst DP, Reggio PH. Molecular targets of the phytocannabinoids: A complex picture. Progress in the chemistry of organic natural products. http://tinyurl.com/bddh3fvy . Published 2017. (Accessed 29 December 2022).
33. Cannabis (marijuana) and cannabinoids: What you need to know (no date) *National Center for Complementary and Integrative Health.* Available at: https://tinyurl.com/4tphvps5 (Accessed: 11 May 2024).
34. Merz, B. (2016) *How to moisturize your skin, Harvard Health.* Available at: http://tinyurl.com/54r97jvp (Accessed: 12 July 2023).
35. Effect of storage conditions on the potency of cannabinoids in cannabis *trimmings* (2022) *Anresco Laboratories.* Available at: http://tinyurl.com/563emzmp . (Accessed: 17 January 2024).
36. Maioli C, Mattoteia D, Amin HIM, Minassi A, Caprioglio D. Cannabinol: History, Syntheses, and Biological Profile of the Greatest "Minor" Cannabinoid.

Plants (Basel). 2022;11(21):2896. Published 2022 Oct 28. doi:10.3390/plants11212896

37. National Center for Biotechnology Information. *PubChem Compound Summary for CID* 5315659, Cannabigerol. http://tinyurl.com/5eed24cb . (Accessed July 4, 2022).
38. Beadle, A. (2021) Cannabichromene: The overlooked cannabinoid, *Analytical Cannabis*. Available at: http://tinyurl.com/mt33w7fu (Accessed: 11 June 2023).
39. Antinociception definition & meaning. Merriam-Webster. http://tinyurl.com/4uf8m4m2 . Published 2022. (Accessed 5 December 2022).
40. Hoover, P. (no date) THCV: Everything you need to know, *CannaMD*. Available at: http://tinyurl.com/275t7vrv (Accessed: 16 June 2023).
41. Hurley EN, Ellaway CJ, Johnson AM, et al. Efficacy and safety of cannabidivarin treatment of epilepsy in girls with Rett syndrome: A phase 1 clinical trial. *Epilepsia*. 2022;63(7):1736-1747. doi:10.1111/epi.17247
42. Wang X, Lin C, Wu S, et al. Cannabidivarin alleviates neuroinflammation by targeting TLR4 co-receptor MD2 and improves morphine-mediated analgesia. *Front Immunol*. 2022;13:929222. Published 2022 Aug 10. doi:10.3389/fimmu.2022.929222
43. Zamberletti E, Gabaglio M, Woolley-Roberts M, Bingham S, Rubino I, Parolaro D. Cannabidivarin Treatment Ameliorates Autism-Like Behaviors and Restores Hippocampal Endocannabinoid System and Glia Alterations Induced by Prenatal Valproic Acid Exposure in Rats. Front Cell Neurosci. 2019; 13:367. Published 2019 Aug 9. Doi: 10.3389/fncel.2019.00367.
44. *Cannabivarin* (2023) *Metabolon*. Available at: https://tinyurl.com/bdhpy9j2 (Accessed: 11 May 2024).

45. Sommano SR, Chittasupho C, Ruksiriwanich W, Jantrawut P. The cannabis terpenes. *Molecules* (Basel, Switzerland). http://tinyurl.com/yc4ywwb8 . Published December 8, 2020. (Accessed 29 December 2022).
46. Cox-Georgian D, Ramadoss N, Dona C, Basu C. Therapeutic and medicinal uses of Terpenes. *Medicinal Plants: From Farm to Pharmacy.* http://tinyurl.com/bded5mpy Published November 12, 2019. (Accessed 22 December 2022).
47. Surendran S, Qassadi F, Surendran G, Lilley D, Heinrich M. Myrcene-what are the potential health benefits of this flavouring and aroma agent? *Frontiers.* http://tinyurl.com/5n9x3fc4 . Published June 9, 2021. (Accessed 29 November 2022).
48. Zhou J, Azrad M, Kong L. Effect of limonene on cancer development in rodent models: A systematic review. *Frontiers.* http://tinyurl.com/3yhjnfry . Published October 1, 2021. (Accessed 15 October 2022).
49. Salehi B, Upadhyay S, Erdogan Orhan I, et al. Therapeutic Potential of α- and β-Pinene: A Miracle Gift of Nature. *Biomolecules.* 2019;9(11):738. Published 2019 Nov 14. doi:10.3390/biom9110738
50. Forest Bathing. *Global Wellness Institute.* http://tinyurl.com/pb9bpm25 . Published September 15, 2022. (Accessed 29 December 2022).
51. Bennett P. What is humulene and what does this cannabis terpene do? *Leafly.* http://tinyurl.com/556e7cva . Published July 28, 2020. (Accessed 29 September 2022).
52. Harada H, Kashiwadani H, Kanmura Y, Kuwaki T. Linalool odor-induced anxiolytic effects in mice. *Frontiers.* http://tinyurl.com/y72fac9r . Published September 25, 2018. (Accessed 15 October 2022).

53. Camphene. *Leafly.* http://tinyurl.com/5n8pzz82 . Published December 10, 2020. (Accessed 20 November 2022).
54. Article S. Benefits of cannabis terpenes: Terpineol, Valencene, and Geraniol. *Leafly.* http://tinyurl.com/muds78np . Published July 28, 2020. (Accessed 29 November 2022).
55. Our favorite 28 terpenes for cannabis products. *Kaycha Labs.* http://tinyurl.com/3sar36dk . Published November 26, 2021. (Accessed 29 November 2022).
56. Editors W. Carene. *Weedmaps.* http://tinyurl.com/jzsaj6vk . Published June 20, 2022. (Accessed 29 November 2022).
57. Carene: A unique terpene with anti-inflammatory & bone-healing properties - RQS blog. *Royal Queen Seeds.* http://tinyurl.com/ywz6sw9r . (Accessed 29 November 2022).
58. Beta eudesmol. Beta Eudesmol - an overview | *ScienceDirect Topics.* http://tinyurl.com/yc4mah63 . (Accessed 20 December 2022).
59. Singh SK, Shrivastava S, Mishra AK, et al. Friedelin: Structure, Biosynthesis, Extraction, and Its Potential Health Impact. *Molecules.* 2023;28(23):7760. Published 2023 Nov 24. doi:10.3390/molecules28237760
60. Terpene of the week: Pulegone. Terpene of the Week: Pulegone: Matthew Mintz, MD, FACP: Internal Medicine. http://tinyurl.com/3zxuczba . (Accessed 15 December 2022).
61. Team BF. What is pulegone? *Botany Farms.* http://tinyurl.com/7ed552ut . Published August 5, 2021. (Accessed 15 December 2022).
62. Terpene Tuesdays: Everything you need to know about sabinene hydrate flavor, fragrance, and Benefits (no date) *Certified Testing Labs: Cannabis, Hemp, CBD, Kratom & Mushrooms.* Available at:

63. Cedrene. *Leafly*. http://tinyurl.com/hr2mwxwd . Published February 3, 2021. (Accessed 20 December 2022).
64. Everything you need to know about Farnesene and its benefits. (no date) *Trulieve*. Available at: http://tinyurl.com/446tddc7 . (Accessed: 03 July 2023).
65. Cedrol. National Center for Biotechnology Information. *PubChem Compound Database.* http://tinyurl.com/2ue6tsbw . (Accessed 29 December 2022).
66. Panche AN, Diwan AD, Chandra SR. Flavonoids: An overview. *Journal of nutritional science*. http://tinyurl.com/tbf7vymk . Published December 29, 2016. (Accessed 29 December 2022).
67. Flavonoid Friday: Everything You Need to Know About Cannflavin A Flavor, Fragrance, and Benefits | *ACS Laboratory*. http://tinyurl.com/yc2cneky . Published 2022. (Accessed 29 December 2022).
68. Yang L, Gao Y, Bajpai VK, et al. Advance toward isolation, extraction, metabolism and health benefits of kaempferol, a major dietary flavonoid with future perspectives. *Crit Rev Food Sci Nutr*. 2023;63(16):2773-2789. doi:10.1080/10408398.2021.1980762
69. Chen AY, Chen YC. A review of the dietary flavonoid, kaempferol on human health and cancer chemoprevention. *Food Chem*. 2013;138(4):2099-2107. doi:10.1016/j.foodchem.2012.11.139
70. Flavonoid Friday: A Guide to Quercetin Health Benefits, Foods, and Effects | *ACS Laboratory*. http://tinyurl.com/yfabwarz . Published 2022. (Accessed 29 December 2022).
71. Flavonoid Friday: Everything You Need to Know About Apigenin Flavor, Fragrance, and Benefits | *ACS*

72. Ashrafizadeh M, Bakhoda MR, Bahmanpour Z, et al. Apigenin as tumor suppressor in cancers: Biotherapeutic activity, nanodelivery, and mechanisms with emphasis on pancreatic cancer. *Frontiers*. http://tinyurl.com/463wrxfc . Published August 5, 2020. (Accessed 29 December 2022).
73. Flavonoid Friday: Everything You Need to Know About Chrysin Flavor, Fragrance, and Benefits | *ACS Laboratory*. http://tinyurl.com/4s2j8hht . (Accessed 29 December 2022).
74. NCI Dictionary of Cancer terms. *National Cancer Institute*. http://tinyurl.com/yc4nfrz7 . (Accessed 20 December 2022).
75. Chrysin. National Center for Biotechnology Information. *PubChem Compound Database*. http://tinyurl.com/mrb7xycx . (Accessed 29 December 2022).
76. Stompor-Gorący M, Bajek-Bil A, Machaczka M. Chrysin: Perspectives on contemporary status and future possibilities as Pro-Health agent. *MDPI*. http://tinyurl.com/3kdhsdm6 . Published June 14, 2021. (Accessed 29 December 2022).
77. Flavonoids Friday: Everything You Need to Know About Baicalin Flavor, Fragrance, and Health Benefits | *ACS Laboratory*. http://tinyurl.com/3vvesbys . (Accessed 20 December 2022).
78. Flavonoids Friday: Everything You Need to Know About Luteolin Flavor, Fragrance, and Health Benefits | *ACS Laboratory*. http://tinyurl.com/4fr4c8dj . (Accessed 20 December 2022).
79. Flavonoid Friday: Everything You Need to Know About Fisetin Flavor, Fragrance, and Benefits | *ACS Laboratory*. http://tinyurl.com/3md5y52k . (Accessed 20 December 2022).

80. National Center for Biotechnology Information. *PubChem Compound Summary for CID* 5281614, Fisetin. http://tinyurl.com/56vuts4x . (Accessed July 15, 2022).
81. Ferber SG, Namdar D, Hen-Shoval D, et al. The "entourage effect": Terpenes coupled with cannabinoids for the treatment of mood disorders and anxiety disorders. *Current Neuropharmacology*. 2020;18(2):87-96. doi:10.2174/1570159x17666190903103923

www.ingramcontent.com/pod-product-compliance
Lightning Source LLC
Chambersburg PA
CBHW070644030426
42337CB00020B/4151